*Health Work
with the Poor*

Health Work with the Poor

A Practical Guide

CHRISTIE W. KIEFER

Rutgers University Press

New Brunswick, New Jersey, and London

Library of Congress Cataloging-in-Publication Data

Kiefer, Christie W.
    Health work with the poor : a practical guide / Christie W. Kiefer
        p.   cm.
    Includes biographical references and index.
    ISBN 0-8135-2776-7 (cloth : alk. paper). — ISBN 0-8135-2777-5
    (pbk. : alk. paper)
        1. Poor—Medical care—United States. 2. Poor—Health and hygiene—
    United States. 3. Medical personnel and patient—United States. I. Title.
    RA418.5.P6 K54 2000
    362.1'086'9420973—dc21   99-045961
                                                                    CIP

British Cataloging-in-Publication data for this book is available from the
British Library

Manufactured in the United States of America

To Lillian, and to the memory of Leatha, Charlotte, and Irene

CONTENTS

ACKNOWLEDGMENTS

I am indebted to the three hundred–odd students who have taken our courses on poverty and health, for sharing their experiences, concerns, and for their criticisms. This book is very much the product of the thinking of Dan Perlman, who taught me most of what I know about the political economy of poverty. Kira Foster, Mary Sue Heileman, and Martin Bustos have also been important mentors, as have health workers and families of Tegucigalpa, Managua, Querétaro, and Palawan, and the "hill" people of Missouri.

PREFACE

This book grew out of a seminar on poverty and health that my graduate students and I have been teaching at the University of California Medical School in San Francisco for the past nine years. This is a student-centered class and all the participants contribute actively to the learning process. Most of the students are candidates for master's degrees in nursing, but included are first and second year medical students and doctoral candidates in social science as well. They take turns in leading class sessions, they critique the readings, and occasionally they make changes in the subject matter assigned. They submit journals of their impressions and questions throughout the seminar, which we use each year as guides in revising the class readings and format.

This book, then, is the product of many minds. The viewpoint that follows, although presented through the lens of cultural anthropology, is strongly influenced by the viewpoints and needs of the health science students. It is aimed primarily at people who have a practical interest in the subject.

The viewpoint advocated here is essentially that of political economy. Health workers have both the means and the obligation to address the root causes of ill health among the poor, not just the symptoms. These root causes are overwhelmingly social and political, and the work of healing at its best includes advocacy. Some readers may see in this book an indictment not only of the American health care system, but of many other institutions that affect the poor. Many Americans hold the view that we live in a land of economic and political equality—a land where the anguished or angry voices of the poor deserve a skeptical response at best. I know of no one, however, who has actually lived and worked among the poor, or studied the vast social scientific literature on poverty in the United States and accepts the dominant definition of the situation. It is not unusual for people with personal experience of poor people's reality to make the indictments found in this book. I only hope that the critical view presented here is in some way constructive.

As for my qualifications in writing about the poor: Most of the ideas in this book come from my reading and from interaction with others who have tried to understand poverty. (Since this book is meant to be more of a practical guide than an academic treatise, I have avoided heavy use of footnotes, preferring to say something about my intellectual debts in this introduction.)

Since the 1960s when I received my doctorate at the University of California in Berkeley, I have had a strong professional interest in social class. This may be a result of my own background: My mother, although a college graduate, came from an Irish working-class milieu, and some members of that milieu have drifted in and out of my life. My father, by contrast, descended from a well-to-do German-American line of professionals, board chairmen, burghers, and even petty aristocrats. For whatever reason, I have continuously studied the ethnographic literature on social class, including many of the excellent ethnographies of the urban and rural poor produced by other anthropologists, sociologists, social activists, and journalists. I have been especially influenced by the works of Carol Stack, Oscar Lewis, Philippe Bourgois, Elliot Liebow, Herbert Gans, Michael Young and Peter Wilmott, Carl Withers (a.k.a. James West), Lillian Rubin, and Jonathan Kozol.

In 1980, when I was teaching courses on the adult lifespan at the University of California Medical School in San Francisco (where I still teach), I felt the need for better studies of social class effects on life span personality development. I spent a year's sabbatical in the Ozark Mountains of southeastern Missouri, interviewing working-class people of three generations. What I learned about poor people's attitudes toward work, self-reliance, and male/female relationships as well as the economics of survival and self-respect in a poor rural setting was invaluable.

In 1993 I was teaching courses on the political economy of health, and I felt the need for more personal experience in non-U.S. working-class settings. I acquired a rudimentary knowledge of Spanish, and spent six months working with a community-based health program in the squatter ghettos of Tegucigalpa, Honduras. Here my main lessons had to do with the way these same issues (sex and gender, pride, and the economics of survival) play out in a different cultural and economic setting. Since then, I have supplemented my cross-cultural experience with a few weeks of study in Nicaragua, Mexico, and the Philippines.

For the past six years I have been a board member of a community clinic serving a low-income clientele in Alameda County. In addition to studying the administration and budget of the clinic, I have spent many hours talking with staff, providers, and patients (who make up a majority of the board also), attending staff meetings, supervising student interns, and observing work in the clinics.

This book falls into three parts. The first part, comprising chapters 1 through 3, addresses the relationship between the health worker and the low-income client. The goal is to help students come to grips with their feelings about working with the poor, and to arrive at an assessment of their role as healers that will make effective action easier. Chapter 1 deals with this relationship at a philosophical level, delving into the question of what is meant by "poverty," how most people react to the poor and why, and how social inequality affects the healing relationship. Chapter 2 addresses the health worker's feelings of alienation from the poor. Using ethnographic accounts, I try to show how many of the "problematic" behaviors of low-income clients result from rational or at least understandable adaptations to insecurity, isolation, and disrespect. Chapter 3 discusses some practical ideas for improving the health worker's effectiveness and efficiency in working with low-income clients. Ways of quickly identifying both material and behavioral resources and obstacles to wellness as they relate to social class, gender, and ethnicity are presented.

Part 2 moves from relationships and feelings to social analysis.

The goal is to help the student understand the historical and political context of poverty in America—the causes and consequences of inequality in our midst. This is particularly important for health workers whose co-workers, acquaintances, and family have little knowledge or sensitivity about the subject, and tend not to support one's interest in it. Chapter 4 looks at the economic and demographic trends that contribute to the kind of poverty we find in the United States today. Chapter 5 discusses current political rhetoric vilifying the poor in order to reduce public support. Chapter 6 focuses on specific health problems of the poor as well as factors of behavior, environment, and access that impair the health of the poor. Planning strategies by health services to improve the situation are also discussed.

Having slogged through the dismal realities of neglect and misunderstanding that characterize health care for the poor, students are usually hungry for good news. Part 3 looks closely at a historically effective strategy for addressing the root causes of ill health among the poor: community organizing. Chapter 7 discusses the evolution and functioning of a community-based health care center for the underserved. Socially conscious health workers see here an inspiring story. Chapter 8 draws together my own and others' experience of trying to facilitate social change. In addition to my own action research in Honduras, Nicaragua, and the Philippines, I draw heavily on the work of activists Richard Couto, David Werner, and Ernest Stringer, and on the literature and videotapes produced by the Highlander School in Newmarket, Tennessee. I have also had the good luck to have personal contact with many activist health care workers through my classes.

Included in each chapter is an "Exercises and Study Questions" section. There are also appendices on internet resources for the study of poverty and on ideas about how to teach health workers in a way that promotes social awareness and activism. The book is meant to be useful both as a textbook for courses on poverty and health, and as a primer and manual for individual health workers serving the poor.

*Health Work
with the Poor*

PART I

Through the Telescope

CHAPTER 1

Encountering Poverty

Poverty: The Absence of Community

For at least a century, the word *poor*, referring to economic status, offers English speakers a double set of images and standards: On the one hand we have the *deserving poor*, people who simply do not have the freedom or ability to work. On the other hand we have that troubling group who could support themselves well enough if they had the moral strength to do so (Katz 1989).[1] This double image has everything to do with America's inability to cope with the problems of its poor people. If we accept the duality, we automatically get trapped in unproductive arguments about who to help, and when, and we never get around to addressing the root causes of poverty itself. We never even consider the question of what poverty is. I begin this book by rejecting the deserving/undeserving dichotomy, by rejecting the notion that poverty is essentially a matter of personal responsibility. The definition of poverty I offer allows us to confront poverty as a social problem, but this is not the only reason I offer it. I think my definition is closer to what most of us really mean when we speak of poverty.

The words *poverty* and *the poor* sound as though they refer to simple realities, and they are often treated that way in popular discussion and the media. Officials, politicians and scholars readily talk about rates of poverty, or poverty trends, as though discussing something as straightforward as tax revenues or school attendance. In reality of course, the words are highly charged with emotion and political opinion, and their meaning is a bitterly contested issue. Some opinion makers portray poverty as a kind of self-inflicted pathology, and the poor as an alien people. Liberals often see the line that separates most poor from the average person as a fuzzy one, and remind us that families cross this line in both directions all the time. Attempts by scholars of poverty to bring order to our understanding of its complexity are not very successful. Their work is undone by politicians who try to win votes by convincing their listeners that poverty is something simple and that politicians know what to do about it.

Understanding poverty and our attitudes toward it require that we consider its history. Social values and economic conditions change, and so do some details of our images of the poor. Yet some of our attitudes are remarkably stable over time. We now look back with horror at the common nineteenth-century practice of putting poor people in prison. Today the poor are kept in squalid housing projects in dangerous slums instead.

To begin to clarify the concept, let us start with the meaning that probably first comes to mind: poverty is "an inadequate command over resources relative to needs" (Oster, Lake, and Oksman 1979, 4), meaning the lack of sufficient money income to regularly purchase basic necessities—food, shelter, clothing, medical care, education, transportation, and so on. This definition has its place in U.S. society, first because most people do need a certain inflow of cash to get by, and fall into serious trouble when they do not have that inflow; and second because statistics on income (though often misleading) are easy to get. Accordingly, the U.S. government tries to identify the poor by picking a certain dollar income level, or *poverty line*, below which people would have a hard time surviving (currently $8,240 for an individual, and $13,880 for a family of three). The number of persons falling below this income line (currently thirty-six million) is probably the most widely used statistic on poverty in the United States today.

However, at once we see difficulties with this definition. For one thing, it fails to take into account other resources that vary from family to family, and that greatly affect the amount of cash income needed for survival. This definition ignores debts, like mortgages and car payments, and fixed assets, like houses and land. It ignores unpaid services, like the frequent chores people do for their families and friends; and noncash transactions of all kinds, like the lending of tools or furniture, the handing down of things no longer needed, and swapping without the exchange of money. It ignores environmental qualities that help or hinder survival, like crime rates, climate, and the distance one has to travel to work, to shop, or to see a doctor. This definition ignores personal qualities, like mental and physical health, knowledge, and charm; and perhaps most importantly, it is blind to the size, loyalty, and wealth of one's social networks. Because of all these things, some people fare far better on a given cash income than others.

If we were able to come up with a more sensitive index of access to basic material needs than income, would we then have an ironclad definition of poverty? I think not. Our understanding of poverty has a moral, emotional dimension that goes beyond mere survival. I think most people would agree that someone can be poor even if they are reasonably well fed and clothed, and free of disease. Isn't a well-nourished inner city family poor if the adults cannot find work, the children's schools are unsafe and ineffective, their housing is frightening and disgusting, they endure frequent insults from persons who disrespect their condition, and they have no prospects of changing their situation? Franklin Roosevelt touched on this moral dimension in his 1937 inaugural speech, when he included the opportunity to better one's life as a basic human need (Oster, Lake, and Oksman 1979, 7). I also think most people would agree that others would be considered less poor than this family, even if their sources of food and shelter were less secure, provided that these others did not yearn for any other way of life, and were not idle, disrespected, or oppressed. Such others are not as hard to find today as you might suspect. These others live in small, well-integrated communities all over the world.

Obviously, our understanding of poverty is undergirded by ideas of decency, fairness, and peace. This understanding has to do with the availability of these absolute moral necessities, and takes into account not only the condition of the people themselves, but of their surroundings as well. We understand that people have the right, not only to survive, but to live in a way we think of as fully human. We have an idea of a normal level of security, comfort, and respect; and that is the level the poor have a right to enjoy also. For some to go hungry while others daily eat their fill of delicacies is an ugly injustice; and the same is true for other basics: the feeling of belonging, of being respected, of sharing with one's fellows whatever life has to offer. Georg Simmel, one of the founders of modern sociology, wrote: "[O]f all the social claims of non-individualistic character based on a general quality, it is that of the poor which most impresses us. Laying aside acute stimuli, such as accidents and sexual provocations, there is nothing such as misery that acts with such impersonality, such indifference, with regard to the other qualities of the object and, at the same time, with such an immediate and effective force" (1909, 19). Whereas misery of other sorts (physical pain, grief) is often inflicted by forces beyond human control, poverty often arises from the unfair distribution of resources. It is one thing to believe that poverty is an unavoidable result of differences in fortune, ability, and locale—it is another thing to believe that it should be tolerated unnecessarily. The great social critic George Bernard Shaw understood poverty as a moral category. His best known play on the subject, *Major Barbara*, proposes an ethical dilemma in which the evils of poverty and war are compared—and war comes out morally superior!

The details of this intuitive moral judgement vary from era to era, from culture to culture, and from person to person, but I think to some extent it is a human universal. We are a social species. We evolved in groups where individuals worked together and shared what they had. To the extent that we are willing to recognize one another's common humanity (an important qualification, as we shall see), we cannot comfortably ignore others' suffering. Recognizing another's humanity is not just compassion for the less fortunate. This recognition also includes a sense of alarm when we see around us an absence of the sentiments that make collective human life endurable—trust, generosity, the easy recognition of our common origins and common fates.

Our willingness to help the "deserving poor," then, does not beg for explanation. But what about the concept of the undeserving? If the perception of poverty is the instinctual perception of a moral wrong, why do most modern societies define a group of people whose poverty is tolerated? In chapter 4 we will examine why, in a historical and sociological sense, poverty persists in the United States. Here, I am concerned with the apparent philosophical contradiction: poverty is by definition something morally intolerable, and yet we tolerate it. To be sure, the philosophical and the historical problems are intertwined, but there are practical reasons for discussing them separately. The former is a problem for self-examination; the latter for social action. To address the former, I am going to focus on three features of industrial society that I think help to explain the prevalence of poverty in the face of universal aversion to it. These are (1) the cultural limits of community; (2) the we/they reflex, and (3) the management of the status quo.

Why Poverty? Urbanization and the Cultural Limits of Community

The social scientific use of the word *community* has a long history and is hard to express concisely. There is a good deal of argument among scholars about whether, and under what circumstances, the concept is even useful. I will use it here because I believe that as an ideal type, that is, as a sociological concept that might not actually be found in its pure form in the real world, the idea of community is extremely useful in understanding the origin and nature of poverty in our society.

As an ideal type, then, community refers to a small group of people living most of their lives close to one another, sharing a common language, history, set of beliefs, behaviors, lore, and values. People in such archetypal communities are thought of as having little freedom of individual choice, since their lives are transparent to their neighbors and since there are so many shared expectations and norms governing behavior. On the up side, resources such as labor, capital, and goods are supposed to be shared through an elaborate set of traditional obligations and rights, and this gives people a certain security, both material and psychological.

This ideal type of community is often used as a theoretical contrast with another ideal type—that of the city. The idea of a city, especially in the United States, is that of a place that brings together in one neighborhood people of diverse backgrounds and beliefs, and where there is a high turnover of residents. As contrasted with those in rural communities, city people tend to work away from their homes, and their jobs tend to be highly specialized, so that there is little shared knowledge about work. The urban setting depends upon monetary exchange, not customary exchange. Services performed collectively in traditional communities tend to be performed in cities either by impersonal bureaucratic agencies (schools, police departments, and so forth) or by commercial businesses. As a result of all these things, city dwellers may know little about each other, and may have very diverse ideas about how to live. The interactions of neighbors are regulated less by custom than by choice, and they may or may not choose to help or even be civil to each other.

It would be a mistake to conclude that community and justice are the same thing. In small communities where people have grown up together, one usually finds a strong sense of belonging that unites people within kin groups and social classes. One usually finds well-developed patterns of mutual cooperation and reciprocity that keep misery within bounds. But in most of these communities one also finds inequalities of wealth and power, and sometimes these inequalities are seen by the poor themselves, as well as by the outside observer, as quite unjust and injurious. In the Southern United States until very recently, blacks and whites were neighbors in small towns and shared a common culture; but it was a culture in which rights and privileges were determined on the basis of race, a rule enforced by violence if necessary. Substituting the word *caste* for race, the same was true for centuries in much of India. In Latin America, a mestizo background played a similar role, and so on.

Behavior between social unequals is to some extent cultural.

It is mediated by learning. In the course of growing up in a given culture, we are rewarded when we show compassion in certain ways, and not in others. We learn by observing our elders when to act on—or even recognize—our feelings and when not to. As anthropologists say, we learn the rules for cooperation, trust, and compassion, along with thousands of other rules for other emotions and behaviors. In traditional societies, inequality is generally seen by the more affluent classes as being a natural and unavoidable state. Poverty is accepted by them as something decreed by powers greater than their own; and the poor themselves are thought to have their own sources of happiness and satisfaction.

The Enlightenment in the West challenged these ideas to some extent, and its dictates of equality have now affected social thinking and law in every urban society. The notion that all humans are created equal plays a major role in government and jurisprudence throughout the world. But cultural learning is never consistent, logical, or unambiguous. Cultures evolve slowly, in response to the accidental conditions of the times. They are not deliberately and rationally designed. They have momentum and inertia, and do not respond readily to changing conditions. Once a belief or practice has ceased to serve its purpose, it takes generations for it to fade away. Besides, culture is simply unable to mediate all the conflicting demands people make on each other in the course of everyday life. As a result, life in even the simplest and most homogeneous culture is full of contradictions. Take the example of the virtue of loyalty. In most cultures, people are urged to be loyal to their conscience, to their parents, their spouse and children, and their employer. In many situations, what may be loyal from your mother's point of view may be disloyal in the eyes of your husband or employer. How often does the average person have to make painful and risky choices as a result of these contradictions?[2]

In small communities, then, people tend to know whom they can and cannot trust, and what they can and cannot hope for. There is sometimes a major change in the political climate of the wider society—the Civil Rights Movement of the 1960s, for example—that leads to new relationships. But failing this, people tend to evolve a workable culture that keeps relations between individuals and classes stable.

There are indeed areas in modern American cities where life resembles in many respects this model of a small community. This is especially true of areas where immigrants from more traditional cultures make up a large portion of the population—ethnic neighborhoods, if you will. The Japanese in San Francisco (Kiefer 1974), the Italians in Boston (Gans 1962), and the Cubans in Miami (Stepick and Grenier 1993) blended in their own ways the traditions of their ethnic origins with the constraints of their urban milieu. But the social characteristics of the city can be seen as major contributors to many of the problems of the urban poor. Urbanism has effects that can greatly aggravate the problem of inequality by allowing social classes to become isolated and mutually opaque. The anonymity and mobility of urban society greatly reduces the knowledge people have of each other. This makes it more and more necessary for the urbanite to rely on abstract, general principles in more and more dealings with more and more others. Under the circumstances, the contradictions within our system of abstract values often have the effect of alienating us from one another.

In American culture, compassion for the unfortunate is a strong abstract value; but this value often conflicts with the other major values of equality and personal autonomy and responsibility. It is a cultural rule that every healthy, competent adult shall be assumed to have the same gifts of intelligence, character, and strength. Such adults should be allowed to choose their own goals and make their own decisions, and should be held responsible for the results of their choices.

When we are speaking about strangers, and not kin or neighbors, the following cultural rules or understandings apply: To help someone who has not asked for help, or to require someone to offer help unwillingly, are both violations of others' autonomy. To ask for help is to admit a shameful weakness; to offer it when it is not asked is a form of arrogance. To help those who could help themselves, even if they ask, is to insult their integrity. To classify a person as needing help is to violate the principle of equality.

Because of the decline of community that can accompany a certain kind of urbanization, even people of the same class know less and less about each other; and those of different classes become even further alienated. Because of this alienation, the structural contradiction between compassion and autonomy in our culture creates powerful ambivalence about suffering. Ambivalence is usually a painful feeling, since it robs us of the ability to act. Observing someone's life, we sense, "here is poverty," and we wish it were not so. If we are middle class, we consider various actions that might change the situation, such as providing charity or make-work, voting for more jobs and better wages, or becoming a social worker. If we are poor ourselves, we consider extending whatever personal help we can afford—sharing necessities, sharing work, joining a cooperative group, advocating or protesting on behalf of others.

But any of these actions is likely to provoke a moral dilemma: Can I truly say that this particular poverty that I am witnessing just now is the result of conditions beyond the control of those involved? Will the good gained by relieving their suffering more than offset the evil done by violating the principles of equality, autonomy, and responsibility? Unless I am fairly sure, I am not likely to act. Worse yet, whatever our own social class, these painful questions discourage us from engaging the poor as ordinary people, and their problem as a soluble one. Rather, the moral murkiness around the topic puts us off. We react defensively to it, we feel guilty about this defensiveness, and we justify it by distancing ourselves from the poor, by invoking the we/they reflex.

Compare our attitudes toward the undeserving poor with our attitudes toward the sick. If someone is in obvious pain, weakened, or in danger of death, there is little moral ambiguity about helping. Life is more important than freedom and dignity. The affliction might be the result of willful self-abuse or recklessness, so that even the caretakers of the afflicted might say that the illness is deserved. But the norms of our culture rule that the self-afflicted has the same right to care as the blameless victim. Because the victim's life is in danger, or he is robbed by his affliction of his abilities, he is removed from the class of equal and autonomous persons. The victim's responsibilities are also reduced. He must try to get well as best he can, including giving up his freedom to those better able to heal him, but even if he fails to do this, he doesn't completely lose his right to be helped. The patient may even bring on his own affliction again and again without losing this right.

To say that a person is poor in itself implies no such shift from freedom to deserving help. Only the helpless, the deserving poor, make the switch. The relief of poverty in the abstract is a social imperative like the relief of sickness and injury; but questions of how to help and whom to help immediately break down into a debate over causes. This debate, between the rugged individualists who hold freedom to be a greater good than charity, and the communitarians who see the greater injustice in the persistence of poverty, has become so much a part of our national life that we have trouble thinking about poverty in any new way.

Judging by my students' and my own feelings, then, most Americans—affluent and poor alike—feel compassionate toward the poor in a general, abstract sense. Statistics on the abundance and depth of poverty in America arouse their indignation. But when confronted by a particular example of poverty—an individual, a family, a slum, a request for help—they tend to feel not just compassion, but also anxiety. They often handle this anxiety by thinking about how they might be different from these people, and wondering whether any action would really help.

Why Poverty? The We/They Reflex

When I was living in Japan, I found it odd that Koreans are the victims of all kinds of subtle discrimination there. After all, Koreans look exactly like Japanese to me. But my Japanese friends could point to someone in a crowd, and say, "That person is Korean." They could not explain how they knew, but they were certain about the judgment. At the time I doubted their accuracy; but as I have observed myself over the years, I have come to accept it. All normal human beings can tell, probably at an early age, from a distance, in an instant, whether or not someone seen in passing is a member of a particular, familiar cultural group. American or European? African American or African? As children we do not as yet know the labels, but as adults we use subtle cues of dress, grooming, facial expression, posture, gesture, and gait to make such distinctions. Not only can we do it with uncanny accuracy, we find it almost impossible not to do it.

Each of us can manage to make ourselves feel sentimental

from time to time about abstractions like "we Americans," or even "we humans"; but we do so by extending our kinship and friendship feelings to cover a larger fantasy-family of "people like us." Only a handful of saints have managed to sustain such feelings for humankind when confronted with the reality. The natural thing for us to do, and as I said we do it unconsciously and without effort, is to make distinctions between us (meaning ourselves, our loved ones, and other people very much like us) and them (everybody else).

Politicians try to make use of our tendency to extend our fellow feeling to abstract entities like nations, but it can backfire. Although his administration marked a high point in social reform legislation, Lyndon Johnson was unpopular in his last years as president. With his heavy Texas accent, he used to begin every speech with the words, "My fellow Americans . . . " For millions who found his policies in Vietnam horrible and his accent strange, his attempts to establish kinship with this opening cliché helped to destroy his credibility.

The well-known psychologist and humanitarian Erik Erikson coined the word *pseudospecies* to describe this phenomenon, the universal tendency to act as though the concept human only applied to the people we personally care about and as though our morals and feelings did not apply to the others. Homo sapiens evolved in small hunting and gathering bands, probably of a few dozen individuals. Each of these bands was likely in competition with other bands for food and territory. Along with all the rest of our mental equipment, we developed in the course of eons the abilities to (a) care deeply about a small number of other people (usually a couple of dozen); (b) recognize immediately the slightest distinction between people from our group and those from other groups; (c) feel wary, if not hostile, toward outsiders.

This we/they dividing line is very emotionally real to us. To the extent that we are left to our unexamined feelings, people on the we side of the ledger really do tend to become for us the only ones worthy of human feelings, while people on the they side tend to become members of another species—one of inferior value and sensibility, to be treated at best as targets of our self interest, and at worst as pests to be eliminated.

Like moral ambiguity, the we/they reflex is made much more serious by the decline of community; and because of this the suffering of the urban poor tends to be far worse than the suffering of those in small, stable communities. While still believing in neighborliness in the abstract, the urbanite—rich or poor—unconsciously adopts the habit of putting people *in general* on the they side of the equation unless some very good reason not to is found. This has been tested by sociology experiments, in which rural and urban people are asked for help by strangers. Sure enough, rural people, whose surroundings are peopled mainly by acquaintances and kin, tend to be much more open and helpful than their city counterparts. They have less of the habit of holding people at a distance, or of suppressing their natural inclination to get involved.

There is an additional dimension to the we/they reflex when it applies to relationships between social classes, a dimension that I will take up in detail in the next chapter. It is that being poor makes it difficult for people to live by the rules of mainstream society. In order to get their basic needs met, poor people often have to adopt ways of life that are unfamiliar, and even unacceptable, to their nonpoor contemporaries. In other words, in the process of adapting to their situation, the long-term, or "hard core" poor often become different enough from others in their appearance and behavior that the we/they reflex is evoked in their relations with the nonpoor. Importantly, it is usually evoked on both sides, each economic class feeling equally uncomfortable in the presence of the other. Since health care encounters typically involve cross-class interaction, it is important for health professionals to understand this.

Classroom discussions about poverty reveal these tendencies clearly. My students and I are easily outraged by reports of the way our society first creates poverty, and then mistreats the poor. But when we are confronted with a poor person, our automatic reaction is to put that person as far as possible out in the they category—to assume that everything about him, from background to character to present style of life, is unimaginably different from our own. This automatic reaction, which we can examine and modify with effort, serves several purposes. It helps us deal with our confusion about what moral response is appropriate. It eases the guilty realization that our own relative affluence is partly due to luck. And it helps us deal with the fear that our luck might run out one day. Poverty, then, evokes sympathy in the abstract, but aversion in the concrete. This is a serious problem for health professionals.

Various interactions of mass industrial urbanism and the we/ they reflex can be delineated by comparing the United States with societies where communities and neighborhoods tend to be stronger, like Norway and Japan. Both these relatively homogeneous nations have much more equitable ways of managing resources than we do. They have lower unemployment rates, far less substandard housing, better medical care, better public transportation, and a higher and more even quality of public education than we do. They may have lower levels of cynicism as well. Both countries have much lower crime and civil litigation rates, higher voting rates, and higher rates of personal savings than America. Having spent considerable time in both countries, I believe that Norwegians and Japanese find it far more difficult than we do to invoke the we/they reflex in their dealings with people of their own communities, and that this encourages them to view social evils as shared problems, even at a national level.

In the next chapter, we look more closely at the lives and experience of the poor themselves. One of the most obvious features of that experience is their overwhelming isolation from nonpoor society. It is not just a subjective feeling. The poor in our society are isolated geographically, economically, educationally, and experientially, to the point that we are actually forcing them to become different from us—to become the others of our guilty and fearful fantasies.

Why Poverty? Mass Society and the Management of the Status Quo

The third important reason for our failure to deal with poverty has been discussed by every liberal thinker from Rousseau to Foucault. It is the tendency of social elites—those who benefit most from existing arrangements of wealth and power—to secure the complicity of society as a whole in maintaining those arrangements.

An obvious example of this tendency is the fashioning of laws by the elite, and the complicity of the poor in enforcing these laws. The American system of property, taxation, and election finance laws produces wildly irrational and destructive gains for the rich, and protects these gains against redistribution. (One percent of America's population owns 37 percent of our national wealth. Ninety percent of our people compete for 14 percent of our resources [Barlett and Steele 1992].) More subtle but no less important is the control of public discussion about the extent, nature, and causes of economic inequality, and the management of public images of the poor.

In the absence of religious or cosmological explanations of inequality, the maintenance (and intensification) of social inequality is made much easier by the decline of community. As our knowledge of each other becomes more and more impersonal and indirect, we depend more and more on the channels of mass communication for our attitudes and beliefs. Even a casual look at the way information and persuasion flows through public channels (TV, press, movies, and so on) in America reveals that a small (and shrinking) homogeneous group—the economic elite—is allowed to control this flow to an astonishing extent. When journalist Ben Bagdikian wrote *The Media Monopoly* in 1983, most of America's major media were owned by fifty giant corporations. By 1992, this number had shrunk to twenty (Bagdikian 1992, ix). Not surprisingly, the mainstream media have a tendency to help construct, and then pander to, public stereotypes of wealth and poverty that encourage a high tolerance of economic inequality.

Images that accompany discussions of poverty tend to depict unmarried mothers and their children, African Americans, the unemployed, and homeless people. The bias in selecting these images appears when one looks at the statistics. In fact, the age-sex group with the lowest average income in the United States is neither young women nor children, but women over sixty-five. Less than 30 percent of America's officially poor (with cash incomes below federal poverty guidelines) are African American.[3] The officially unemployed (those registered with employment agencies) head about one fourth of families with official poverty incomes; and the homeless make up only about a sixtieth. Rather, these images are selected to appeal to the need of the majority (who fit none of these image categories) to distance themselves from the poor and to feel morally superior. They offer an image of the poor as promiscuous, idle, nonwhite, and ragged.

In case people still feel guilty enough to want a generous welfare system, the media also embellish the idea that public support may be too generous already. Having imaged the poor as people on public assistance, they regularly report pronouncements on the high cost of welfare programs, and rarely mention, for example, that all income payments to the poor amount to less than 10 percent of the federal budget, and are shrinking. Rarely is there serious discussion of what it might actually cost to provide sustainable jobs for the unemployed, decent wages for the underpaid, decent housing for the homeless, or decent health care for the uninsured.

Media images of the rich are not particularly flattering, since news about their crimes and follies makes especially interesting reading. On the other hand, there is even less useful information available to the public about the rich than about the poor. They enjoy the privacy that money can buy, which is considerable. When privacy fails, they have public relations experts and lawyers to help control what is said about them. Do you know your local gentry's income or where it comes from, or how they spend it, or what they own, or where they got it, or what boards they sit on, not to mention what they do all day? (In egalitarian Norway, at least local newspapers regularly report how much money the richest people in their area make—to the penny.) On the other hand, when our rich want to speak to the public, they have access. In addition to owning the media, or having friends who own it, they are its chief customers—they decide how advertising money is spent. Access and privacy go hand in hand to ensure that their opinions, but not their identities, abound in the media.

Health Work and the Poor: The Ideal of Equality

Ingmar Bergman's widely acclaimed film *Wild Strawberries* is about an elderly doctor, Isaac Borg, who is searching for meaning as he enters the twilight of his life. Like many people his age, Dr. Borg is given to nodding off at odd hours, and he has plenty of time to dream. Many of his dreams are nightmares, in which his habitual views of himself are challenged, point by point. In one of these nightmares, he visits himself taking an oral exam from an arrogant young man who seems certain of his incompetence. The opening question: "What is the first duty of a physician?" To his horror, Dr. Borg finds himself completely at a loss to answer. "The first duty of a physician," sneers his tormentor, "is to ask forgiveness!"

An insightful dream, on a point American health care has almost forgotten. For over a century prior to the 1990s, certain physicians and ancillary people in health care (health insurance, hospital administration, medical and pharmaceutical research and manufacturing) relentlessly sought, and won, increasing power over their patients and society. The leaders of this movement must have been those—probably a minority in their professions—who held the naive but popular belief that scientific knowledge is superior to all other forms of knowing, including the kind of intuitive wisdom that forms the basis of all moral and spiritual systems. The physician community, made up as it is of purported scientists, is above control or criticism by those whose knowledge is merely spiritual, social, or political. Western biomedically trained doctors share with the physicist or chemist two crucial features: their work is indispensable in a modern society, and their knowledge is superior to any layperson's who might have an opinion about their work. This superior knowledge applies to the social uses of their science as well.

Some time ago, in the midst of a research project in the Korean American community, I happened to have an attack of lower back pain. After several remedies failed, I found my way to an acupuncturist well known in the Korean community. Standing in his tiny apartment in a poor section of Chinatown, he asked me in Japanese (I spoke no Korean, he no English) to describe my trouble. He listened carefully, but made no comment. Instead he knelt on the floor, placed a stick of incense in a censor in front of him, lit it, and sat silently with bowed head for ten minutes. Then he rose, and relieved my back pain in ten minutes with acupuncture. I paid him twenty dollars. I knew little about his religion. I didn't know what his ritual meant to him, and if I had I would probably have found it quite strange. But looking back, I am sure his act of humility had much to do with the success of his treatment. By placing both of us in the position of supplicant, he dramatized our equality "before God," or as a humanist would say, "as frail and ignorant but worthy beings." At that moment, I was entirely ready to be healed by him.

The point that the leadership of American medicine seems to miss is that the practice of medicine consists of humans caring for humans—an ethical equality of subject and object—and this makes medicine morally distinct from physics and chemistry. Physicians need not dramatize their own frailty in order to heal; but if they deny that frailty, they run the risk of becoming complacent. A medical organization that denies the ontological equality of patient and healer can end up failing in its fundamental mission of letting the needs of the patient, and not those of the physician, guide every aspect of its work. The first duty of physicians is to ask forgiveness, for their dreadful challenge of fate.

We are now seeing the social results of just such an institutional denial of medicine's essential humanity. The moral failure of our health care system has become so obvious that even the industry's spin doctors can no longer conceal it with a steady output of medical miracle stories. The relationship between power, knowledge, and virtue turns out to be another of those areas of cultural self-contradiction where values clash and outcomes are always ambiguous. On the one hand, there is nobility in any profession dedicated to the relief of suffering; and there is honor in mastering a complex body of knowledge and skill. Health care is often a gripping drama, in which the dedication and ability of the professional is pitted against the irrational evil of disease and death. On the other hand, the health worker often assumes a pose of superiority over patients and others, who must obey, or suffer the consequences—a potential violation of our belief in the freedom and dignity of the individual. To justify others' faith, the provider occasionally feels compelled to act on blind instinct, challenging fate to expose (sometimes disastrously) the overstepping of her limits.

Accordingly, health profession training constantly strives for certainty, trying to push back the boundaries of doubt and lighten the burden of moral anxiety borne by the Dr. Borgs of the world. But this very struggle paradoxically increases the guilt of the provider. As technology and knowledge increase the range and fatefulness of the choices available, the risk, and the pain, of those choices grows. With the power to manipulate fertility, prolong costly and painful incapacity through lifesaving measures, or predict genetic disaster in a couple's longing for parenthood, the dilemma of the provider grows to monstrous proportions. Finally his fate is like that of a leader in a deadly war, weighing the use of hellish weapons in the uncertain pursuit of peace.

Every health provider knows that the more vulnerable the patient is, or the more dependent the patient is on the decisions of the provider, the more likely is the abuse of medical authority, and the more serious its consequences. Vulnerability and dependence are directly related to lack of power, which not only includes lack of physical and mental capacity, but also lack of status, influence, relevant knowledge, and wealth. At any level of health, the poor, as we have defined them, are likely more vulnerable than the nonpoor. Their choice of providers or treatment options, their ability to question or influence others' decisions or seek redress for mistakes, are all likely diminished by their poverty.

There is now an extensive literature in medical ethics that addresses such issues. Veatch's widely used text, for example, urges both physicians and patients to use a "moral point of view" in their relationships—a point of view in which each respects the other's autonomy: "If I were a patient I would want . . . " and "If I were a physician I would want . . . " (Veatch 1982; quoted in Freeman 1987, 374). I don't know what the average health professional's awareness of medical ethics is, or how many agree with Veatch's prescription; but even if the position were universally accepted and conscientiously followed, it would not in my opinion entirely solve the problem of inequality that I am addressing. In addition to the principle of patient autonomy, there must be knowledge on the provider's part of the constraints—material and psychological—on that autonomy that are imposed by the very nature of any relationship between a relatively affluent and powerful person and a relatively poor and powerless one.

In getting to know the residents of the South Bronx, Jonathan

Kozol (see chapter 2) learned that few of them ever escape the appalling conditions in their neighborhood hospitals by seeking care in Manhattan institutions, even though they are eligible to do so. They explained to him that they don't feel welcome outside their own neighborhood, that they don't match the Manhattan surroundings, and feel disrespected there.

In seminars with student dentists at UCSF, I often hear anxious stories about the hostility of some of their patients—usually poor people on Medicaid. These patients seem to mistrust the students, the office staff, or even the faculty; and they handle their mistrust by taking a combative attitude toward everyone and everything. These same patients often miss appointments and fail to follow instructions for self-care. Many are unhappy about the results of their dental care.

Even if the poor were a uniform group psychologically, I could not claim perfect empathy with them, but having been interested in how various kinds of poor people see the world, and having looked for answers both in personal discussions and in literature, I can say one crucial thing about the way poverty affects relations between patients and health providers: Being poor makes many people feel vulnerable, helpless, and inferior in many situations; and seeking care is often one of those situations.

It would be hard to exaggerate the importance of this from a health standpoint. If you think about what good health is, how it is different from ill health, you will understand that good health, however you define it, depends on feeling effective and worthy. Staying well is one thing. Getting well is another. The return to health is usually helped when the patient trusts the provider and himself enough to believe in the treatment and follow instructions. When such feelings are constantly undermined by reminders of helplessness and low worth, recovery suffers accordingly.

Promoting the health of patients, in other words, depends to some extent on restoring and maintaining feelings of power and worth. But because of the power inequality that separates the health professional and the low-income patient, these feelings of helplessness often come to the fore during health care encounters where the poor are involved. Knowing this, many health workers make special efforts to compensate for the vulnerability of the poor.

They donate or discount their services, they cost-shift, they innovate cost savings, and they work under inferior conditions in order to serve low-income clients.[4] Although commendable in intent, this is usually futile in the long run. It can actually make the situation worse, by replacing autonomous self-care with dependency on services that are unsustainable and given with an air of patronage that undermines the ability of individuals and communities to value their own resources.

There is no way of absolutely eliminating the ill effects of medical power. They are to some extent inherent in the act of caring. That is why I call it a paradox. All providers who work primarily with the poor know or should know the importance of minimizing those ill effects through sensitivity to their clients' vulnerability. But I would like to suggest a further dimension of self-consciousness that is now rare among health providers. The obverse of the power equation also holds. Health care practice is less paradoxical, and closer to the ideal of a pure service, when the power of the provider and the patient tends toward equality. There are many things health care workers can do, when working with the poor, to promote this ideal situation—and later on in this book we will consider some of them. But what is one's responsibility?

Obligations of the Health Worker

I was once asked by a local civic service group to help organize a public symposium on international health. Two on the panel were physicians well known for leading top-down medical missions in which teams of American doctors selected poor communities overseas for brief sorties of intensive clinic work. Two other speakers were strong advocates of the bottom-up approach—capacity building in local communities, which could then sustain better health by improving their control over such resources as land, water, housing, and work conditions. In the midst of the symposium, one of the medical mission doctors strode to the podium and vehemently denounced the bottom-up people. He called them "prostitutes," and said that they should be prohibited from polluting medicine with such ideas. He spoke against health professionals taking part in any political activity, saying that it was not only beyond medical expertise, but a violation of the health worker's oath of moral neutrality.

The host organization seemed embarrassed by the exchange, and I regretted not having warned them. That exchange exposed one of the major dividing lines in the health professions—between those who strictly hold that the job of the health care provider is to understand disease and treat the individual patient, and those who also include in the job the understanding of ill health and the treatment of the patient-in-the-world. For the former, the private settings of consultation room, laboratory, and bedside dictate professional ethics; for the latter, health care is also practiced in the board room, the legislature, the courthouse, and the street.

I cannot resolve this argument for everyone, but here is my own view. I have said poverty is not the simple lack of means to survive, but the morally painful fact of unnecessary suffering imposed by those with resources on those without—a fact that makes us uncomfortable by our very nature as a social species. From this I draw four conclusions. First, as human beings, we deny our nature when we ignore poverty in our midst. Second, inequality is a social as well as a personal fact; it is as much the result of collective customs and laws as of individual habits and abilities. As a members of a particular society, we all share responsibility for the social causes of poverty in that society. (I will return to this point in chapters 5, 6, and 8.)

Third, health is one of the basic resources whose unfair distribution defines poverty. The health professional has greater access than others to information about the distribution of health and health care, and greater influence than others in affecting that distribution. Moreover, the distribution of health services is affected by, among other things, the cultures of the health professions— what skills are taught and how, what rewards await what kinds of work, where resources are located and who has access to them. But the individual health professional does not have to accept the canons of her professional culture blindly; she herself contributes to the shaping of that culture.

Fourth, poverty contributes to the inequality of power that separates the provider from the patient. As such, it helps to obscure the fundamental ethical equality of their relationship. This in turn leads to false values and distorted standards throughout the health professions—fee structures and logistic barriers that restrict access; mentoring that produces self-centered career goals; technology that serves the few at the expense of the many and creates painful ethical dilemmas instead of relieving physical suffering. This same inequality undermines the individual provider's ability to restore health with the help of the patient's feelings of effectiveness and worth.

All these considerations should take their due place in decisions about the importance of the social, versus the personal, approach to one's work.

Exercises and Study Questions

1. What are some well-known literary treatments of poverty? How are the poor portrayed in these fictional works, and why?

2. When you see the words, *the poor*, what is the first image that comes to mind? What feelings are associated with this image? What are some sources and consequences of culturally shared images?

3. Have you known someone who had a poverty level income but was not poor?

4. What criteria other than cash income would you use to measure poverty?

5. Discuss your personal experiences of the we/they reflex.

6. How does your status as a health professional give you power, prestige, and authority? How do you use these resources?

The Poor in the Mirror

CHAPTER 2

Why Get to Know the Poor?

Throughout most of this book we look at poverty from a broad social perspective. We ask not so much why a particular person is
poor, or what we as individuals can do to help this person; but
rather how social forces produce and sustain poverty, and what
actions might address these forces. Meanwhile, however, working
with the poor is for many of us an everyday personal experience,
and often a stressful one, not an exercise in social philosophy. Few
things are more frustrating to a health professional than to feel sure
you can help a certain patient, but you can't seem to get the patient to cooperate. This happens with all kinds of patients for all
kinds of reasons, but it happens more often when professional and
patient hold different assumptions about some key aspect of the
situation, and neither one knows just what those assumptions are.

In this chapter I address this problem as it applies to communication between health professionals and their low-income clients.
I do this by facing our guilt (an important emotional complication
in working with the poor); reminding us that we can respect people
without being like them, that a healer and a poor patient's lives
are usually very different, and their assumptions are often likely
to be different as well; and by offering an interpretive framework
that the health worker can use to build up a picture of her clients'

assumptive world—a picture that should improve communication between them.

In chapter 1 we tried to understand the paradox of our tolerance for poverty in our midst, in spite of our aversion to it. I am reminded of William Faulkner's observation (in "A Rose for Emily") that people "cling to that which has robbed them." Perhaps we cling because the robbery so injures our feelings that we cannot look at it directly, and not looking, we cannot see it for what it is. Viewing poverty from the corner of our eye piques our feelings of guilt (for not being poor) and fear (of being poor); and we quickly look away. It is a Medusa that turns the gazer to blind, inactive stone. We are ready to be told that it is not really there, or that its presence is normal and not really an offense at all, or that it is temporary and will soon be cleared up.

We can begin by looking more closely at ourselves. As long as we fail to act we are not entirely innocent; but neither is our inaction something easy to overcome, kept in place as it is by the contradictions of our culture and the limitations of our energy. Having seen this, perhaps we will give ourselves room to take small steps. Here I suggest one such step: to view the Gorgon's head again—through the mirror of ethnography and narrative journalism.

Looking at the actual lives of the poor, as they have been reported by ethnographers and journalists, is for me extremely difficult. I do it because, like bitter medicine in small doses, it allows me to confront my anxiety a little at a time, and in the process, to draw courage from my gradually expanding knowledge. What I say in this chapter cannot be a substitute for reading the first-hand accounts I drew on. If you lack direct experience, you will have to read the works I cite—Kozol, Kotlowitz, Bourgois, Stack, Lewis, Howell, Fitchen, Couto—for yourself. The most important message of their work cannot be summarized in a textbook, because it is the experience of the humanness of the poor, and of the pain they feel, which can only come (if you do not stay long among them yourself) from reading the words of the poor themselves.

In what follows, I have two objects. The first is to help those health workers who need to unfreeze their ability to engage the poor with energy and creativity. The material in this chapter should make poverty more familiar to them, and less of a frightening chimera. Second, I want to help health workers fashion their own mental tools for engaging poor people in mutually helpful ways. In order to do this, I have artificially reorganized the accounts of the ethnographers into sections covering human needs—security, love, respect, stimulation, and meaning. In chapter 4, I go over some of the same ground, differently organized according to the perceived social problems attending poverty—especially idleness, unwed pregnancy, and violence.

The Politics of Explanation

"I am prepared to say to the poor, 'You have to learn new habits. The habits of being poor don't work'" (House Speaker Newt Gingrich, quoted in *The New York Times*, June 16, 1995).

There are as many different ways of being poor, and of coping with poverty, as there are ways of being nonpoor. The usefulness of social science comes from its effort to sift what is orderly and predictable from all this variety, so that the practitioner, or philosopher, can begin with a set of testable propositions, a logical map of the terrain, in trying to understand her own experience.

To perform this service on the subject of the poor, we have to focus on the more-or-less predictable effects of poverty on human nature, but in doing so we are immediately caught in a dilemma. If we present the lives and characters of the poor as inherently systematic and subject to discoverable rules, we imply something about the causes and remedies of poverty. We imply that the internalized rules or systems we are proposing somehow cause the phenomena of poverty, and that changing these rules—that is, changing the attitudes and practices of the poor themselves—may get rid of the problem. On the other hand, if we say that the principles that order the lives of the poor are strictly external and situational—that is, political and economic—we imply that there is really nothing that can be done at the level of personal relationships between individual helpers and individual poor persons or families (except organizing for political action, which, by the way, I have no quarrel with). Either of these implications can become a political position, generating policy about how to improve society. This is exactly what has happened as a result of scholarly attempts to systematize knowledge about the poor, as we shall see in the next two chapters.

The easiest way to deal with this dilemma is to ignore it, to take sides and say either that the causes of poverty are located within or beyond poor families and communities. I find I cannot take this way out. While I believe that structural conditions like job and housing discrimination, ghettoization, criminalization, and the incestuous relation between wealth and political power must change if resources are to be distributed more justly, I also believe that health workers can help to ease the stress on individual clients if they have a picture of how those clients' individual experiences and behaviors are necessarily, or at least predictably, shaped by access to resources. But I want it to be clear that by presenting the lives of the poor as systematically affected by their circumstances—as to some extent inherently understandable and predictable—I am not suggesting either (a) that the poor are a homogeneous culture, or (b) that social reform should be directed at the minds and bodies of the poor themselves.

Who Are the Poor?

So who are *the poor*?

- The poor are people who want the same things every other human being wants, but whose access to many, or all, of those things is somehow systematically restricted.
- All human beings want to be secure, loved, respected, to have excitement and stimulation, and to experience life as purposeful and orderly.
- Every society has certain general rules about how these things should be pursued.
- Every human being encounters difficulties in getting these basic needs met in the approved ways, but the poor have special difficulties because of their restricted access.

In a complex, affluent society like mainstream America, the "proper" pursuit of basic needs takes a lot of material and social resources and knowledge. For example, to get basic needs met an adult usually has to do socially approved work—have a trade or business, hold a job, or run a household. In order to do any of these, a person has to have quick access to information, reliable transportation, housing, health care and hygiene, and, usually, formal education. One also has to know the rules that go with the work.

For a majority, being loved and respected in the proper way also involves having a stable, monogamous marriage. To this end, a person must have a reliable income and be able to solve the myriad problems and challenges of intimate relationships, such as the maintenance of mutual trust, the settlement of disagreements, and the joint planning of long-term goals. Women are expected to fulfill themselves through the raising of children, a craft that today proves highly challenging even to affluent couples, let alone the socially and economically marginal. Access to socially approved kinds of excitement (travel, sports, the arts, "an exciting job") also requires knowledge, social skills, and usually, money.

If we look at the poor as people who have systematic, long-term difficulties in meeting their needs in a socially approved way, we can understand a great deal about them. The most important insight from this exercise is to see how being poor systematically isolates people from mainstream society, thereby deepening their poverty. Widespread concern over the behavior of the poor can be seen as a reaction to the nonstandard or unapproved ways poor people go about fulfilling their needs, given their lack of means to do things the mainstream way. Most poor people have to rely on others in similar straits for sociability and support, and thereby come to share certain common ways of doing things. A vicious circle develops, in which the disapproval nonpoor people feel for the habits and lifestyles of the poor provokes an avoidance of the poor—as friends, employees, customers, co-workers, schoolmates, neighbors, even casual acquaintances. This avoidance results in the isolation of the poor, which of course contributes to the difficulty they have in pursuing socially approved lifestyles, thereby widening the gap of difference and indifference.

In what follows, my goal is to narrow this gap by clarifying specific differences between mainstream, "acceptable," strategies for getting one's needs met, and the kinds of strategies that typically evolve in poor families and neighborhoods. Since there is no standard list of human needs in the literature on human behavior, some readers will not be satisfied with the list (security, love, respect, stimulation, and meaning) I will use, but that matters less than whether my list serves the function of making the lives of the poor more intelligible. Elsewhere (Kiefer 1988, 188–205) I have written extensively about where I obtained this list.

Several problems arise from using a functional model (the fulfillment of basic needs) for understanding behavior. First, it implies that most behavior is somehow explainable in terms of universal, more-or-less rational motives—something that cannot be demonstrated. Second, it implies that we can infer those motives reliably from what people do and say, which is at best a shaky assumption. Third, it requires us to set aside some of the complexities of the relationship between behavior and purpose. For example, the purpose of a behavior often depends on its meaning for the actors, and meanings are overlapping, intertwined, and subject to frequent revision. Finally, it is highly artificial to divide behavior up by motive, since almost all human acts serve a variety of purposes at the same time. Libraries have been written by anthropologists on such problems; but those libraries serve different aims than the one I am pursuing.

The Pursuit of Security

Cecil (thirty-five) lives in The Flats with his mother Willie Mae, her oldest sister and her two children, and his younger brother. Cecil's younger sister Lily lives with their mother's sister Bessie. Bessie has three children, and Lily two. Cecil and his mother have part-time jobs in a café and Lily's children are on aid. In July of 1970 Cecil and his mother had just put together enough money to cover their rent. Lily paid her utilities, but she did not have enough money to buy food stamps for herself and her children. Cecil and Willie Mae knew that after they paid their rent they would not have any money for food for the family. They helped out Lily by buying her food stamps, and then the two households shared meals together until Willie Mae was paid two weeks later. A week later Lily received her second ADC check and Bessie got some spending money from her boyfriend. They gave some of this money to Cecil and Willie Mae to pay their rent, and gave Willie Mae money to cover her insurance and pay a small sum on a living room suite at the local furniture store. Willie Mae reciprocated later on by buying dresses for Bessie and Lily's daughters and by caring for all the children when Bessie got a temporary job. (Stack 1975, 37)

After [her partner's bicycle business failure] Julia had to sell her furniture to support the family and they were turned out of her room for not paying the rent. Julia's *comadre*, who lived [in a nearby apartment complex] permitted them to sleep on the floor of her kitchen until they could find another room. Eventually the *comadre* moved out, and they took over her place for a hundred pesos. With Julia's earnings they bought second-hand furniture and once more had a home. Julia provided the food and clothing because Guillermo [her partner] could only be persuaded to take responsibility for the rent and the electric bill.

One day Guillermo saw miniature water bottles in metal stands on sale in a toy market. He figured out how to produce them inexpensively and went into business again. . . . With his earnings from the bottles he again bought stolen bicycles and began to rent them out. He also got hold of an old bottle cooler, stocked it with ice and bottles of coke, and went into the soda-dispensing business. To build up his bicycle agency he gave a free bottle of pop to each person who rented a bike. When, however, police inspectors began to investigate all bicycle agencies in an attempt to cut down widespread thefts, Guillermo hastily sold at cost all of his "hot" bicycles. . . . His bicycle agency gone, he also stopped selling soda pop.

To make up for the loss of income he stocked a tray with candies to sell to the neighborhood children and continued to service bicycles. . . . Besides this he collected empty bottles and broken glass and gathered and bought up scrapwood. A friendly watchman at a nearby government warehouse gave him small quantities of wood and sawdust on the condition that he would not sell it. But he did secretly sell it and once or twice a week he would also exchange a large bag of sawdust for a few pounds of meat from a local butcher. (Lewis 1959, 142–143)

These two examples of the subsistence strategies of two poor families were chosen because they make the same point in very different ways. The first comes from a northern U.S. urban neighborhood of African American migrants from the rural South. The barriers these families face to full economic participation are chiefly their race, their lack of appropriate training for well-paid urban jobs, their residential segregation and lack of transportation, and their historical entanglement in a web of social ties to other poor families that, while it sustains them at times, at times also limits their mobility and freedom of choice. The second example comes from a slum area of Mexico City. More and more Latin American families without the land or capital needed to farm or start a real business, or the education for a good job, settle in large cities either in their own country or the United States. (Mexico City in 1990 had a population of over twenty million, while Los Angeles had a Latino population of 1,391,000—the population in both cities mostly poor like Julia and Guillermo.) They do so precisely because, as densely populated places where others have jobs and wealth, such cities provide myriad tiny (and often illegal) economic niches like those exploited by Guillermo's family in their struggle to survive.

Many other accounts of the lives of poor families tell stories like these of the struggle for subsistence—stories with certain common themes. First, and most important, making a living is precarious for people who are not well tied in to the mainstream economy. In general, poor people have the kinds of low-skilled jobs that are most casually filled and terminated, and therefore do not become strongly integrated into a work team. More than the middle class, they are likely to depend on sources of income (peddling, scavenging, welfare, swapping) and sources of basic needs (housing, food, clothes) that can suddenly fail. Those who are utterly without social prestige, powerful allies, or capital (not all poor) often have their livelihood disrupted by the capricious acts of others, or of their environment, over which they have no control. The mainstream way of making a living usually involves considerable planning, such as saving for big purchases, investing in things that will save money or generate income, pursuing education. With little ability to predict their economic situation from week to week, many poor people simply find that such strategies do not work for them. As Janet Fitchen says, "In the day-to-day living on the borderline between just barely getting by and not making it, the freedom to act quickly—to make changes in family arrangements, to move to a new location, to spend half the food budget on something else—is an essential adaptation to poverty living" (Fitchen 1981, 73).

The penetration of welfare bureaucracies has added a particularly painful aspect to the unpredictability of livelihood for many poor people in the United States—their dependence on impersonal social agencies for basic necessities. In my work among the poor in Central America, I found that people relied almost entirely on kin and neighbors, since there is virtually no welfare system. This sharing of hardship often produces the beneficial side effect of mutually respectful and sympathetic socializing. But recent ethnographies of the poor in America are consistent in the way they report the unfeeling capriciousness, sometimes deliberate, sometimes merely incompetent, of welfare agencies. Although thousands of welfare officials are no doubt sincere and competent, welfare laws are generally written by well-to-do legislators with little interest in the actual experience of the poor, and they are written (as we shall see in chapter 5) so as to enforce—in ways often inappropriate and sometimes impossible—conformance to middle-class norms. They are written in ways that humiliate the recipients. Working in welfare agencies itself is considered low-status work, and employees are often victims of inhumane management policies. Unfortunately, it is not unusual to find those employees resentful of their jobs and shockingly ineffective in their performance.

Mrs. Washington [who has cancer] does not get out of bed when I come in. She seems much weaker than she was during July. When I ask how she feels, she answers, "Better... worse. . . . It comes and goes," then shows me a notice she just received from the company that manages her building. "It's a dispossess. Eviction order." She takes it back and puts it by her lamp. "My rent is paid directly by the city. I don't see the money. When the city's computers make an error, I get one of these. In '92 I got one and it said I had to be recertified. I went to welfare and I told them that I was already certified, so they said, "Okay, you're fine. Two months later, I got the dispossess."

"The problem is they have no continuity. Every other month, it seems, the welfare staff gets fired and my social worker disappears."

When I ask the name of her social worker, she says, "I don't have one. I had one but her husband died and she went back to Puerto Rico. She came by and told me that she wasn't breaking down her caseload since there wasn't anyone to take her place. I still don't have a new case worker." Picking up the dispossess again, she says, "It says I owe $6,000. I got three of these last week. They push them underneath the door. I have to try to get a lawyer." (Kozol 1995, 43)

A nonpoor person can understand the existential quality of such lives in the abstract, and even imagine having to live this way temporarily in a pinch. But what is difficult for the nonpoor to understand is that living with blunt uncertainty like this constantly, year in and year out, requires a mind-set that is fundamentally different from the middle-class one. Adapting to it at the level of survival requires people to keep their minds focused on the myriad immediate and shifting possibilities for, and barriers to, having their needs satisfied. One result of this mind-set is that people who are chronically poor often seem not to see the longer term consequences of what they are doing. Another way of stating this frequent difference between poor and nonpoor is to say that the nonpoor live immersed in a set of assumptions based on the consistency of life and the tractability of the remote future, while many poor live with an opposite set of assumptions. As a result, the nonpoor often view the poor as impulsive, disorganized, unreliable, and self-destructive.

There is one very important exception to the principle of unpredictability in the lives of the poor: reliance on other people, generally kin, neighbors, and close friends. While people of all classes value and cultivate their close social bonds, for the poor these bonds are fundamental to daily survival. The low-income family that cannot count on the periodic help of neighbors and kin is insecure indeed. In the examples above, if Cecil and Willie Mae had not been able to count on Lily and Bessie, they may either have lost their home or gone hungry for some time. If Julia's *comadre* had not let the family sleep on her floor, they would have been out in the street. As a result, the quality of social relationships is different across social classes. Middle-class employers and bureaucrats find it exasperating that a poor person will go AWOL from work or miss an appointment if a kinsman demands his help or company. But this can be seen as a form of long-term planning. For the poor, close relationships are capital, and are often simply more important than other commitments.

The erosion of community, then, which I spoke of in chapter 1, is relevant here. Read any ethnography of a modern urban ghetto, and then of a traditional poor rural town, and you will immediately see the effect of social breakdown and isolation on the economics and psychology of the poor. To be cut adrift from people with whom one shares a common history and understanding is hard for anyone. For the poor it is a form of disaster. This issue reappears again and again in our understanding of the poor.

Taking into account the unpredictability of basic resources in poor communities, then, helps to some extent to explain class differences in behavior. But there is another important piece of the explanation. Although all middle-class people sometimes feel they do not get the respect due to them from certain others, generally they get treated at least as equals by acquaintances and strangers alike. Most have little experience of what it is like to be viewed with contempt by society at large—or even to fear that this is the case. Since Americans put so much emphasis on self-reliance and economic achievement, it is hard for the nonpoor to realize that the poor's need for respect is often even greater than their need for economic security. In short, members of the mainstream find it hard to understand why poor persons would jeopardize their livelihood, or take life-threatening risks, in order to protect their self-esteem. Yet this is often what is happening when a poor person quits a job over a seemingly minor insult, or opts for a lower-paying, less secure, more dangerous, or less legal trade in order to earn the respect of his peers. When I was doing field work in the Ozarks, I met several young men who had quit relatively secure jobs in the city to pursue precarious lives in the countryside, where they could "be their own boss," and do work that was considered fitting for a man—gleaning firewood, hunting small game, fixing cars, and doing seasonal farm work. I will return to this when I discuss respect.

The tendency of men to seek respect in this way is related to yet another important facet of the pursuit of security that separates some poor communities from the middle class: violence. Although the image of the violent ghetto projected by the mass media is overblown, inner city poor in the United States are more at risk of violence from a variety of sources—chiefly armed drug dealers and youth gangs—than the middle class. In some places, like the public housing projects of Chicago and East Harlem and the barrios of Los Angeles, this threat causes many families to live in constant fear. It is hard to say how the fear affects the behavior of these people in other respects, but it must have consequences. If nothing else, it probably contributes to the sense that the future is unreliable, even unreal, and encourages risk-taking over planful living. I will return to the subject of violence in chapter 5.

The Pursuit of Love

The word *love* covers such a broad range of meanings that the observation that people need love is hardly self-explanatory. The best way to clarify what I mean by it is to contrast love with the other human needs. *Security* refers to the feeling that nothing devastating will happen to me in a material sense, that I can count on having what I need to survive, and be free of threats to my physical being. *Respect* means the feeling that other people accept me at least as an equal and accord me at least the same privileges and courtesies as they expect for themselves. *Meaning* refers to the sense that life is not completely arbitrary and senseless, but in some measure understandable, and follows rules that I can accept. *Love*, by contrast, means that my unique personhood—my existence as a separate, irreplaceable being—is valued for itself by someone else. It means that the terrible existential loneliness of being a unique and unknowable consciousness is made tolerable by a bond that requires my presence, my existence as-it-is. It usually, but by no means always, has something to do with kinship or sexuality.

It is hard to write about the pursuit of love among the poor, for several reasons. For one thing, our culture romanticizes and mystifies the topic so heavily that we all have fantastic ideas about it. We Americans expect so much from our love relationships that most of us live in constant pain about them. By the same token, we tend to give respect to others based on our perception of how successful they are at love. To say that a person, or a class of people, have difficulty managing love relationships (usually meaning some idealization of what such relationships should be like) is almost equivalent to saying that they are somehow defective and unworthy of respect—never mind that we ourselves generally fall far short of our own ideals on this score.

In any walk of life, one finds warm families and cold families, loners and extroverts, loyalties and betrayals; but ethnographies of the poor consistently show two things: that love among blood kin, and especially between parents and children, is highly important and usually enduring, and that sexual love between men and women tends to be difficult and brittle. The people in the ethnographies—especially the men—rarely talk about love, and when they do, it is often with ambivalence. What is revealing is the effort and self-sacrifice that go into relationships, especially the relentless efforts of mothers to keep their children safe and secure against tremendous odds. Many poor families and kin groups provide a surprisingly strong sense of well-being and self-respect to their members, as I will discuss again when I turn to the pursuit of respect.

Surprisingly often, the work and worry of love extends not just from parents to children, but from offspring of all ages to parents, to aunts and uncles, even to in-laws. Jonathan Kozol speaks of the relationship between teen-aged David Washington and his mother, who has cancer. They live together in a crumbling public housing project in the drug-infested and violent South Bronx:

On an evening in August, when I'm home in Massachusetts, David calls me around midnight after his mother's gone to bed and asks if we can talk.

I ask him how she's feeling and he says, "I can't get her to eat. She's vomiting and coughing. She keeps waking up at night and going to the bathroom, usually at two or three. . . .

"I keep waking up myself. Even if my mother isn't up, I wake up anyway. I go in her room to see if she's asleep. If she's sleeping I just sit there by her bed." When she's feeling very sick, he says, he stays in her room and sleeps at the bottom of the bed.

"Sometimes in the afternoon, when I come in, I find her crying. I try to get her to talk to me but she won't talk. I know that she doesn't want to make me sad, but when she won't say anything, her being silent makes me sad. She thinks that she's protecting me but she cannot protect me. . . . "

"Last night . . . I got the thought that maybe she's not eating so that she'll be sick enough for SSI. I wondered if she's starving herself so that she'll qualify, so that they'll say, 'This woman's sick enough. She qualifies.'" He doesn't cry but sounds as if he's struggling to control his voice. (Kozol 1995, 22)

Pharoah [age nine] felt sorry for his father and tried to cheer him up. If there was a basketball game on, Pharoah would try to get his father involved. He'd make a gentleman's bet on one team; his father would take the other. Anything to keep his father from becoming too pensive. Then, Pharoah knew, his father would only get depressed. (Kotlowitz 1991, 168)

Love amid scarcity often entails serious sacrifice, and not surprisingly generates strong ambivalence:

Last month the AFDC people sent me forty dollars to get a couch. Instead of getting the couch I took my money over to Mama's and divided it with her. I gave her fifteen dollars of it and went on to wash because my kids didn't have a piece clean. I was washing with my hands and a bar of face soap before the money came. [Washing the clothes] ran me up to six dollars and something with the cab that my sister took back home. I was sitting over at the laundry worrying that Mama didn't have nothing to eat. I took a cab over there and gave her ten more dollars. All I had left to my name was ten dollars to pay on my couch, get food, wash, and everything. But I ignored my problems and gave Mama the money. . . . She was over there black and blue from not eating—stomach growling. The craziest thing is that she wouldn't touch the rent money. . . . She paid her sister her five and gave me five to give the kids something to eat. I said, "What about my other ten?" but she put me off. She paid everybody else, and I'm the one who's helping her the most. (Stack 1974, 35–36)

One of the strongest tenets of mainstream Euro-American culture is that heterosexual love should be synonymous with monogamous marriage, especially on the part of women. It is all right for young men—and increasingly, women also—to "experiment" with sex, but it is generally assumed that the minute youthful romance develops into "true love," the principals should commit to a lifelong relationship. The myth is that romantic love and successful marriage are practically the same thing.

In fact, of course, heterosexual relations rarely get far on romance alone. It is useful as a catalyst to bring people together long enough to get acquainted; but feelings of sexual attraction are too fragile, and distractions too numerous in real life, to create lasting bonds. Those middle-class couples who manage to live together for many years usually do so because they are able to develop a predictable relationship—each partner knows, or feels that they know, more-or-less what the other will do in a given situation, and this creates a feeling of security. Long-term couples know which topics are safe to talk about and which are not; which tastes and opinions should be cultivated and which avoided; and when it is safe to expect sex, work, material contribution (money or goods), nurturance, or understanding. Marriage is largely a matter of trust.

Such relationships of course do occur in poor families as well, but they are even less common than in the middle class. It is simply extraordinarily difficult to develop mutual trust when (a) plans which couples make together, and projects which they undertake, have a low probability of success; (b) commitments of one partner to the other often cannot be kept because demands of others intervene; (c) both partners have experienced a lot of disappointment in relationships with others; (d) both partners have developed the existential style I spoke of above (of making the most of immediate opportunities at the expense of long term goals); (e) strong bonds between blood kin serve as the mainstay of security and companionship; and (f) the self-esteem of one or both partners is compromised, so that they find it difficult to accept or believe in the devotion of another. If a spouse or partner will not commit to a goal the other strongly wants, if they cannot be counted on to fulfill a promise, if the loyalty of each partner to blood kin often takes precedence over the partnership, and especially if they do not consistently defer potentially hurtful feelings and decisions until an agreement has been worked out with the partner, a relationship based on emotional intimacy is not likely to last.

When partnerships between low-income men and women are harmonious and lasting, as many are, one can be sure that they are the result of remarkable patience, determination, and maturity—of a rare capacity to love.

The heterosexual relations of parents are immediately and dramatically passed on to children. In many low-income families and communities, fragile relationships have become normalized in the expectations men and women grow up with, and such expectations naturally tend to be self-fulfilling, as each sex assumes its expected roles. During my field work in rural Missouri, I asked an elderly widow what kind of a man her husband had been. "Oh, he was a *good* husband," she said with satisfaction. "He always worked, he never hit me, and he only got drunk on Saturday nights."

Residents in some poor African American communities seem quite comfortable ignoring the norms of the Euro-American middle class, having found their own residence patterns more satisfying. Men and women often form parental relationships without being married, as evidenced in the community where Carol Stack did her research: "Claudia Williams, who lives down the street from Lily, talked to me about Raymond, the father of her two children.

'Some days he be coming over at night, saying, "I'll see to the ba-bies, and you can lay down and rest, honey," treating me real nice. Then maybe I won't even see him for two or three months. There's no sense nagging Raymond; I just treat him as some kind of friend even if he is the father of my babies"' (Stack 1974, 119).

Among the Euro-American poor, marriage appears to be more important as a marker of status, and I think this helps to account for a certain amount of domestic discord. Many women hold the stereotype of men as irresponsible and often predatory and vio-lent; and men reciprocate that women are impulsive and manipu-lative. Yet it is marriage, nuclear household, and children that really establishes maturity for both sexes. These dynamics make career planning difficult, and one common result is that people tend to conceive children "by accident" at an early age first, then marry, hoping that their union will work out "against the odds." Some-times it does.

Interwoven with the complex dynamics of sexual love is of course the matter of having children. The pride surrounding the birth of children and grandchildren, and the affection that is lav-ished on small members by poor families, are legendary truths. They are truths that often puzzle, even anger, nonpoor observers, who wonder how such people can rejoice at the prospect of more mouths to feed. The middle-class world, with its emphasis on in-dividual autonomy and achievement, tends to focus at once on the tremendous responsibilities of parenthood. An environment ar-ranged for the maximization of its potential is taken to be the birth-right of every child. We react with indignation to the idea that the primary function of children might be to give status, love, and se-curity to their parents and kin; that their right is simply to share whatever little a loving family can spare.

But this formula makes better sense within the political economy of the poor. Here children often represent one's only chance to leave any kind of a legacy or to make one's parents proud. Here the parent-child dyad is the one relationship where sustained mutual love seems guaranteed. Here security in old age is almost synonymous with parenthood. Here hope of success can only be founded on starting life anew. Here children are among the rare tokens that one is, or once was, desired. Where the motivation to keep one's own life going day after day can take more will than ordinary people have, children often are the only thing that provides that motivation. Perhaps it is the middle-class parent's desire for children that needs explaining.

In this discussion of love, I have not touched on relationships among friends, or among close-knit networks found in churches and voluntary organizations of all kinds. In any social class, such relationships can be extremely close, enduring, and nurturing as well.

The Pursuit of Respect

There may be circumstances where poverty itself is no cause for shame, but in the United States of the 1990s such circumstances are hard to find indeed. The American myth is that anyone who really tries can make it on his own. Not just being economically poor, but having the physical and social markings of poverty—a dialect, a skin color, an educational or work background—is enough to consign one to a disrespected position in mainstream society. As I mentioned in the discussion of security, those who have little difficulty getting respect have trouble understanding what a consuming concern it can be when it is widely withheld.

If you listen carefully to the way poor people present themselves, you can hear some consistent themes in their strategies for claiming respect. One such theme is a complex of self-attributes we can call *toughness/quick-wittedness*. Starting with the facts of economic insecurity and the unpredictability of life I mentioned earlier, poor people often learn quite young, by personal experience and observing their elders, that trying to make and execute long-range plans is likely to be depressing and exhausting. It is better to take the world as it comes, cultivating the qualities of endurance, agility, and guile. There is, after all, a certain heroic quality in these traits. The Biblical Abraham dickered with God over the fate of Sodom, and Homer repeatedly refers to his classic superhero as "Odysseus of the many devices."

There is pride, then, for many poor in their ability to endure and even laugh at hard luck, and to steer their way nimbly through a chaotic life. Again, these gifts often widen the gap between classes, as when health and welfare workers find their middle-class assumptions about foresightedness and honesty disappointed in their dealings with clients. As middle-class life becomes more dominated by the corporation and the bureaucracy, it becomes more predictable and routine, more rewarding of the virtues of reliability and planfulness. I will return to the toughness/quick-wittedness complex below, when I discuss the pursuit of excitement.

Because of the different roles assigned to men and women (and perhaps due to their biology as well, but that's another debate), the pursuit of respect is a very different issue for the two sexes. Both my own experience and ethnography are clear on this. For poor women—at least for those with children—housing, clothing, and feeding their families is an overwhelming first priority. Respect, especially from kin and male partners, is important to most women, but takes a back seat to basic survival issues. The middle-class bias is that self-reliant survival should come first, before "luxuries" such as respect or excitement. Accordingly, I find myself tempted to think of working-class women as more virtuous than their male consociates; and I have to remind myself that my moral biases are not pertinent here.

Low-income men, on the other hand, seem to fall along a continuum on this issue at any given point in their lives—a continuum whose extremes are represented by two types. We might call these the *villager* and the *warrior*. At the villager end are those for whom the searches for respect and for love are closely intertwined—those who identify with a close-knit kin network or political or religious community, and whose feelings of being respected are grounded in this identification. The work habits and social lives of men at this end are almost impossible to characterize. Many place little importance on income, type of work, or relationships with others in their neighborhood or workplace. Many work at low-status, low-paying jobs—often jobs that leave them time to devote to the families or organizations that give their lives meaning. They generally avoid the all-male peer-groups characteristic of the warrior style. I believe the villager way of managing respect is quite common among poor men, but it is an adaptation that is very little known, for obvious reasons. It is an adaptation that rarely causes problems for society, and about which we find nothing bizarre or extraordinary. The life of Mrs. Washington's son David in *Amaz-ing Grace* (Kozol, quoted above), and of Guillermo Gutierrez, the non-*macho* family man in *Five Families* (Lewis, quoted above) may be examples of the villager type. One of Bourgois's East Harlem Puerto Ricans had "made it" out of the crack houses and into the legitimate job world. He had experienced a religious conversion that led him to question the values of his East Harlem peers, and moved to the suburbs. His relations with both his old and his new social environments remained tenuous, emphasizing the difficulty of changing from one culture to another—in his case, from a cul-ture dominated by warriors to one dominated by villagers (Bourgois 1995, 172–173).

The warrior end of the male search for respect we find the rebellious anti-heroes of many studies of poverty. Through this style, men who are discounted by mainstream society (both poor and nonpoor) because of their lack of education, social skills, and ability to perform at "respectable" jobs, become hypersensitive to signs of disrespect. These men often find relationships with lov-ers, authority figures (teachers, bosses, police), and mainstream society in general painful and hard to manage; and their adapta-tion is to cultivate values of toughness, independence, and indif-ference to norms.

Herbert Gans (1962) referred to this style as the "action seeker"; and Joseph Howell (1973) called it "hard living." In its milder form, the warrior style is simply *macho*—quick to enhance one's sense of masculinity by dominating women, children and other men, and by avoiding situations (like menial work or egali-tarian sexual bonds) where one feels weak. In its more extreme forms, it can extend to dangerous activities like substance abuse, violence, and crime. Coupled with the existential worldview dis-cussed above under "security," the warrior style can lead to the sort of self-destructive behaviors that drive health workers crazy.

Warrior men generally prefer work that gains them respect for strength and courage and where they are their own bosses or are supervised by "strong men" like themselves. Since respect is cen-tral to their well being, they may be surprisingly quick to leave even relatively secure, well-paying work if they are disrespected by employers, co-workers, customers, or themselves while doing it. They tend to be extremely alert to anyone who might challenge their dignity and autonomy, including bureaucrats and officials, ministers, teachers, and health workers. Their wariness of being exploited protects them from many "improvements" and therapies that the middle class would levy on them. Bourgois quotes Primo, one of the East Harlem crack dealers whose lives typify the warrior style:

> If you're young, you're a fucking idiot if you're working.
>
> My boss, she wanted me to go to school, too. Well fuck her, man! I'm here [at the crack house] and I'm working. I want my money.
>
> And they talk about that school shit 'cause they're pampered, and lead pampered lives. Everybody can't go to school a lot. Some people have to live, man. Especially if you got a son, you got to. . . . People got to do things.
>
> I was eighteen then and Papito, my son, was already born. I mean, you want things in the world. You can't wait for some fuckin' degree. (Bourgois 1995, 151)

As the example of Bourgois's religious convert shows, some men switch from a warrior to a villager style (and the reverse is also probably true). Religious conversion is a fairly common form of this, but religion is not necessarily involved.

The Pursuit of Stimulation

A side of human nature that is rarely talked about, but explains a great deal about our behavior, is our constant need to be entertained—a need fundamental to our survival. If you watch the young of any large-brained animal—cat, dog, ape, dolphin, bear, otter, sea lion—you can easily recognize the very human trait, curiosity. The advantage of having oversized brains is that such brains can be quickly and easily programmed to recognize and react appropriately to millions of idiosyncratic details about one's environment. Small-brained types, however, do not have to collect experience in order to round out their behavioral programs—they are born with most of their programming in place. The price of big-brained adaptability is the *tabula rasa* character of the young brain, and with it the necessity of a vigorous desire to be programmed—a hunger for stimulation, the raw material of new information of all kinds. With the exception of a few species, most animals outgrow their curiosity when they reach sexual maturity. But we humans belong to that elite group that also includes dogs, chimpanzees, and dolphins—a group that keeps an intense hunger for programming, for sheer sensory input—throughout life. In fact, one of the worst forms of torture for a human being is stimulus deprivation, such as solitary confinement in a bare, unchanging environment.

The importance of stimulation throughout the millennia of human history has led to an astounding variety of ways to get it. Art, music, drama, sports, hobbies and games, cuisine, architecture, clothing and body adornment, eroticism, humor, gambling, conversation, warfare, ritual, stimulants and narcotics, travel, the "pure" sciences, the humanities, and the industrial arts serve mainly to satisfy our stimulus hunger.

This would seem to imply that life in primitive societies, with simple technology and a small territory, must be oppressively dull. But although you and I might get bored living on the arctic tundra or the Kalahari Desert, I do not think the native inhabitants do, for two reasons. First, primitive people who are well adapted to their environment have an exquisitely detailed knowledge and appreciation of the details, of both their natural habitat and their society, and a rich folklore and mythology about those details. The nonindustrial mind-set infuses every aspect of its world with meaning. The shapes of clouds, small sounds in the night, a subtle track in the snow or sand, a smell, all are as significant as, say, the labels on supermarket shelves are to us urbanites. The primitive person knows to an extent that urban people can hardly imagine the histories and intrigues, family trees, roles, offices, skills and habits of her neighbors. There is much to think and talk about.

Second, human playfulness seems to adapt to the typical levels and types of stimulation we find in our environment. The small stimuli of everyday conversation and work, the change of seasons, the rites of completion and beginning, a slight innovation in a weaving, a particularly good singing voice—such things seem to satisfy when they describe the range of usual experience. People also become inured to the stresses of primitive life. Heat and cold, thirst, hunger, injury and illness with rudimentary medicine, natural disaster—such things are generally handled with tolerable levels of anxiety in simple societies.

The tremendous complexity and range of experience in industrial society, then, may be as much of a curse as a blessing. For one thing, our pleasures are now allocated on the basis of class and wealth. If I think about my own life, for example, I immediately realize that most of my diversions would disappear at once if I were not affluent and well educated: I live next to a broad suburban park where I can safely run and bicycle; I enjoy novel foods and wines; I meet new people with interesting experiences; my work, being professional, is different from month to month and year to year; the view from my house is pleasant; I have a working TV, a VCR, and a stereo; I get new books, CDs, software, tools, clothes, and gadgets; I go to plays, movies, and concerts; I have access to the internet; and most important of all, I have enough control over my life that I can anticipate and enjoy these things with peace of mind. I can even enjoy stressful novel situations, like working in the Third World, because I can leave these situations and return to my comfortable life at will.

Added to the social class bias in access to experience is the socially destructive effect of marketing stimulation for its own sake in industrial society. It is in the interest of consumer industries, and especially of the leisure industries—sports, entertainment and travel—that consumers should be perpetually seeking new, expensive, and ephemeral experiences. Under the circumstances, a culture of excitement develops, where all kinds of goods and experiences are judged increasingly on their excitement value, and people for their ability to give and get stimulation. Another schizophrenic contradiction is introduced into our basically puritanical culture: While on the one hand virtue is identified with self-discipline, efficiency, and attention to simple spiritual values; on the other hand a life without excitement shows a deplorable lack of spirit and imagination. Humorist Will Rogers was fond of saying that he cultivated "all the popular vices."

Aside from those few who still live in isolated rural towns far from the shopping mall, this is the situation in which America's poor find themselves. With resources barely able to meet survival needs, and immersed in a culture of excitement where simplicity is devalued, they must allocate scarce resources between the competing "necessities" of subsistence and excitement.

For many, it is a no-win situation. To the extent that one lives simply in order to be self-reliant, one puts one's poverty on view. To the extent that one allocates resources to the pursuit of pleasure, one draws the censure of the mainstream world for wastefulness and lack of self-discipline. One message that the poor are bound to draw from this contradiction is that they belong to a class that is not welcome to share the enjoyments of other classes. Fitchen (1981, 86–87) describes a rural family that decided, with a social worker's help, to improve their economy by saving diligently to put in a well, so that they would not have to spend many hours a week hauling water. After some months, the social worker returned, and "was surprised and dismayed to see, parked on their front porch, a snowmobile," paid for, in part, by the money that had been put aside for the well. It turned out that an acquaintance had offered the snowmobile to them at an amazingly low price, and, on top of that, had accepted some car parts as part of the payment. The parents felt that this luxury was justifiable, since they were one of the few families in that area whose children did not have access to such a coveted symbol of affluence and source of excitement. But they felt deeply humiliated in the presence of the social worker's shocked anger.

Earlier I spoke of the effects of economic uncertainty on the quest for respect, and outlined the self-image of toughness/quick-wittedness. To some extent this style is cultivated in poor families as a solution to the need for excitement as well. Fitchen, in her study of poor white rural families, spoke of their perception that life is less a series of orderly routines or sequences, and more a sequence of "dramatic, spontaneous events" (1981, 140). In the process of learning that (a) many middle-class sources of excitement are not available and (b) planfulness may be frustrating as a general life strategy, poor children may also learn that a highly unpredictable life has certain entertainments of its own. The excitement of an unexpected opportunity seized, or a disaster averted, can produce a more intense rush of emotion than the slow fruition of a long-term plan. Drug and alcohol use is an obvious corollary of this style.

I think this dramatic existential style of life is also encouraged by the entertainment industry, which both glorifies risk taking and thrives on the patronage of the working classes. In this sense, there is a resonance between the top and the bottom of our social hierarchy: the fictional (and quasi-fictional) adventures of television, movie, sports, and music heroes on the one hand, and many poor people's perceptions of their own lives, on the other.

It should be clear at once that there is potential synergy between this dramatic/heroic perception of life, and the warrior style of respect seeking. Bourgois relates that someone called his Puerto Rican dealer friend Caesar and his kind stupid for not getting regular jobs. Instead of the violent reaction Bourgois feared, Caesar responded with a proud defense of his warrior style, in which he identified with a popular rap singer: "That's right my man! We is real vermin lunatics that sell drugs. We don't wanna be part of society. It's like that record [1990 rap record by Public Enemy], 'Fight the Power!'"

The point of this discussion is not that poor people try to dramatize their lives more than middle-class people do. Although mainstream Americans pride themselves on their self-restraint, one need only think of the quantity of money spent by the middle class on the pursuit of excitement to see through our prudish claims. Excitement (often sexualized) is the main selling point in a vast outpouring of ads for cars, clothes, beer and liquor, tobacco, sports equipment, travel, perfumes and cosmetics (and cosmetic surgery), jewelry, and entertainment. Who buys all that stuff? The point is simply that poverty results in different styles of stimulation seeking, and the class associations themselves encourage mainstream Americans to look with disapproval on the choices of the poor.

The Pursuit of Meaning: Community

The sense that life is pointless, or that the events that shape one's life are random and without order or justice, is one of the most painful human experiences. All human beings have an amazing capacity to believe absolutely in something, and we are strongly drawn to believe in whatever seems to offer a solution to our immediate problems, whether it be a leader, a doctrine, or a private conviction. Some belief systems are so remote from ordinary experience that they appear bizarre to most of us. But crises in belief occur only when there seems to be no doctrine at all, or no course of action, that will satisfy this craving for certainty.

There are many examples in our literature, including the Book of Job in the Hebrew Scriptures, that show how sickness and suffering challenge a person's sense of meaning and justice. We are susceptible to alienation when we are sick, and this susceptibility is itself an additional threat to wellness. We need a sense of wholeness and order more than ever to get well. For this reason, it is especially important for health workers to understand where their patients' sense of wholeness comes from.

From working with the poor, I get the somewhat paradoxical impression that many of them have a healthier sense of life's meaning than most middle-class people. The sheer difficulty of surviving, and helping one's loved ones survive, in a harsh environment seems to give a sense of purpose to the daily activities of many. Perceptions of the self as resilient and determined are strengthened by adversity. While they often question the wisdom of specific official policies and the intentions of specific officials, there is little evidence that the poor are more likely than others to see the world in general as meaningless or evil. I do not fully understand why this is so. Undoubtedly, there are as many ways of understanding the world from the vantage of poverty as of affluence, and one definitely finds advanced philosophers in all kinds of poor communities. But I know of one way in which poverty can actually enhance life's meaning. It is the sense of connectedness to the oppressed of all eras and all places—a sense of sharing the struggles and hopes of one's fellow poor, whether they be the people next door or the exiled Israelites of the Hebrew Scriptures. The suffering of poverty is a distinct feeling, and a very widespread feeling. Shared feeling creates meaning.

One expression of this meaning is in the pride and independence found among poor people who belong to a true community. I found this enviable strength—even serenity—among the residents of the urban shantytowns of Honduras and the isolated villages of Mexico and the Philippines. It has been described in hundreds of ethnographies. In the United States, it is a powerful force in many remote hollows of Appalachia and the Ozarks, and in many black farm villages of the South.

Mattie Lee Holcombe Moorer lives in Lowndes County, Alabama where 62 percent of the residents' incomes are below the poverty line (1970 median income, $2,810). She speaks of the Civil Rights Movement in the 1960s:

> There was fear among people at that time. Yes, Lord! But we were all at a point that there was so much that we were tired of, and we were willing to risk our lives to get to vote and whatever else went with voting. There is a time for everything according to Ecclesiastes 3, and that time had come in Lowndes County.
>
> How was I able to deal with my fear? I was born in Lowndes County, not figuring to go nowhere else to live but Lowndes County. (Couto 1991, 87)

Jesse Cannon Jr. lives in Haywood County, Tennessee (1980 median black income, $2,555—27 percent of national median):

> Let me tell you a little bit about Douglas Junior High School and what it was like. Of course, it was an all-black school. One that had as its teachers people who lived in the community for the most part. . . . They were an extremely proud group of teachers, kids, and parents, and it was one of these schools where the PTA had the community behind it. The community would get together and have picnics and something like this to raise money for the school. . . .
>
> Invariably, when kids from Douglas Junior High School went to high school—at that time they went to an all-black school in Brownsville—they were the class leaders. (Couto 1991, 30–31)

Often in such communities people share more than surroundings and lived experience. They share belief. Robert Mants, also of Lowndes County: "The movement here and elsewhere represented prophetic truth to a lot of people who were motivated by religious beliefs. Contrary to a lot of them being called communist, what inspired them was belief in God. People saw themselves pretty much like the children of Israel in the biblical days" (Couto 1991, 91).

Because poverty is one of the most widespread forms of suffering, and because all religion deals with suffering, religion often has a special vitality among the poor. One of the messages of many faiths—Judaism, Islam, Buddhism, Christianity—is that suffering itself is not pointless, but somehow part of a larger plan, or lesson. We may not understand the lesson at first, but we will in the end if we study it; and it is well worth learning. Jonathan Kozol reports a Christmas sermon in a parish of the South Bronx where the early deaths of AIDS, overdose, and violence are everyday events:

"There were in the same country shepherds abiding in the field," [the minister] reads, "keeping watch over their flock by night. And, lo, the angel of the Lord appeared . . . and they were sore afraid. . . . But the angel said unto them, fear not; for, behold, I bring you good tidings of great joy."

In alternating passages, first in English, next in Spanish, she then begins the text of the sermon she has been working on for several days. The text for the sermon is from the passage she just read: "The angel said . . . fear not."

The fear that the shepherds felt, she says, is a fear that all of us know well in our own lives. "It was not the 40th Precinct. It was not a drug bust. There was no helicopter like the one we saw last week on Beekman Avenue. But people were afraid." . . .

She stresses the simplicity of God's message at Christmas: "The kingdom comes to us in the form of a baby. This little child was born to a poor family. They lived among the cast-offs of society. Because of Herod's ruling that the first-born must be slain, the child was at risk of death from the beginning." . . .

"Look at the children who are here with us tonight," the pastor says. She nods at the acolytes beside her. "Joey dreams of becoming a priest. Anthony wants to be a writer. Every child among us has a precious life and holds a precious dream." No matter how terrifying life may seem, she says, we need to hold fast to the words of the angel and those of the psalmist: "I will fear no evil."

The unassuming character of the sermon seems to touch the people deeply. (1995, 87–88)

The importance of belief, and the way belief is supported by community—shared experience, shared resources, shared values— make the ongoing loss of community, for poor and nonpoor alike, especially troubling. In later chapters the problem of social disintegration is taken up in more detail. Here we note one of its effects. To read the ethnographies of the increasingly isolated and strife-ridden ghettos of Chicago, Washington, and New York, and the dying rural neighborhoods of New England, alongside those of the old close-knit Southern black farmlands, is an enlightening experience. One begins to see how threads and islands of community have been carried from those old farms to the Northern cities. A strong family here, sternly led by a matriarch or patriarch from the old land; a community-wide tradition of exchange there, among a group of people with a distant shared past; a vital church here, led again by elders conscious of an earlier era; a civic organization there, seeking to sow new seeds of trust. But mostly, one sees the numbing alienation and loneliness of young people by the millions, growing up in projects full of armed strangers, encircled by the remote bureaucracies of school, police force, welfare office, and clinic—growing up without any idea of a real community. This is indeed poverty.

Exercises and Study Questions

1. Think about a particular behavioral problem you have encountered working with low-income patients. How might this problem result from adaptation to being poor? What interventions might be most helpful?

2. List the main ways you go about meeting your basic needs for security, love, respect, meaning, and stimulation. How does your economic situation and social class help?

3. What are some procedures and policies of your work place (clinic, hospital, social service agency) that might make access more difficult for poor people? How might some of these be changed?

4. The human need for stimulation is rarely discussed in psychology or medicine. Why do we not pay more attention to it?

5. What major changes have you seen in American society in your lifetime? How might these changes affect the middle class and the poor differently?

The Poor in the Consulting Room

CHAPTER 3

Healing and the Contexts of Health

Whatever their class backgrounds, health workers who look closely at the adaptations of the poor will see the expression of familiar themes. This, I hope, is a step beyond guilt, sentimentality, self-righteousness, or protective intellectualization. As such I believe it is an important step toward greater effectiveness. But in today's health care environment, providers usually work under difficult time pressures. Getting insight into patients' lives and gaining their trust may be necessities for good care, but are apt to be costly necessities.

Poverty as a characteristic of a patient population complicates this problem in many ways. For one thing, the social knowledge base of the health worker and that of the patient are likely to be quite different; for another, their styles of communication and assumptions about the relationship may be at odds. Moreover, low-income patients tend to be sicker when they seek help than the nonpoor (see chapter 6), and, for reasons we have been discussing, they are more likely to miss appointments, to fail to call in, and not to comply with instructions. To be effective at working with the poor, the health professional needs an efficient strategy for cross-class communication.

55

The solution will be different according to the personality and life experience of the health worker, and according to the setting in which one works. Some workers are casual in their style, others formal; some have more personal experience living among the poor than others; some work in settings where they see the same patients repeatedly, or visit their homes; others have only a few minutes of contact before the patient disappears from view forever. The following ideas will not work well for everyone, or in every setting. They are derived from my experience working with graduate nurses and medical students, and observing a variety of health providers working with the poor.

When dealing with patients of our own social class or ethnic group, we automatically draw on a large body of knowledge about the context of the patient's health problem. With a few simple questions drawn from our own experience, generally we can get a rough idea of the patient's physical and social environment, style of life, and values relevant to the problem. If we are good at our jobs, as we gain experience working with a given population our sense of context becomes richer and more accurate, often without our even noticing it.

In other words, the problem we are discussing is largely the result of (you guessed it) living in a complex, urban society where privacy and anonymity are the rule; where social types are segregated; and where mutual knowledge among people is minimal. In the small traditional communities where most people lived in past eras, the richness of shared social, economic, and cultural information was taken for granted.

Take the simple example of knowing the neighborhood where a patient lives. Without hesitation, you know where the patient's home is relative to pharmacies, grocery stores, bus routes, health providers, and other resources. You have a sense of the physical condition of the houses and streets, the degree of safety at various times of day. If you know the area really well, you know which pharmacies and stores deliver, and what their price range is. You know the quality of services offered by health and other agencies.

This knowledge increases your efficiency enormously, in many ways. It helps you establish rapport and trust with the patient, by conveying understanding of his life and empathy for his difficulties. It also helps you to help the patient stay honest: the more you know about a client's background and way of life, the more difficult it is for him or her to manipulate the facts—a survival strategy that sometimes works too well with unsophisticated outsiders. Together with information about the patient's physical condition, culture, and lifestyle, social knowledge also gives you some sense of what kind of treatment plan will work. (Does he drive? Can he read a phone book, a diagram, a prescription label? What foods does he like? What is his knowledge of anatomy? Who are his social supports?)

A Framework for Contextual Knowledge

The more remote the patient's life experience is from our own, the more important it is to systematically acquire a sense of that experience—a sense of the context of the person's health. Of course this takes time and effort, but it may not be as difficult as it sounds. A great deal can be learned with a few simple techniques. Here I propose a framework for getting and organizing contextual knowledge about patients—simply a way of thinking through the task, so that the health provider can quickly inventory what she already knows about a group or person, and identify what else is needed and the fastest way of getting it. Looking at this framework, you will probably see that you already have a good deal of contextual information on many of your patients. The exercise suggested here should help you use that information more efficiently.

Ordinarily, we build up our picture of another person by mentally pasting together information that we have already gleaned from many different sources (which I will discuss in a moment). When we meet people who are like ourselves in class, gender, and culture, or are of a social and cultural type we are familiar with, we already have a good deal of contextual information relevant to understanding them. We either have the examples of our selves, family, friends, etc., or we have built up a fund of ethnological lore, which we fashion into a set of hypotheses about what a patient's life is like and what to expect from him; and we base our conduct on these hypotheses.

As we get to know a particular person well, we refine and

adjust our hypotheses about his social, physical, and biographical contexts, and these refinements get added to our store of information about "people like this"—they modify our stereotype, you might say. At the same time, we are picking up bits of contextual information by talking with other people of the same gender and type, by reading and seeing films about them, or visiting neighborhoods where they are concentrated, and so on, and we add this information to our assumptions about the contexts of his experience.

Contexts: Class/Culture, Service Area, Gender, and Person

To systematize this natural and automatic process a bit, let us divide our information about patients into four main contexts: the context of the social class and ethnic group, the context of the service area or neighborhood, the context of gender, and the context of individual biography. This is somewhat arbitrary, and we could use other organizing contexts, like region, age, or family—but we want to keep it simple. Most of us who have passed through the American education system are quite familiar with this way of organizing social knowledge, and some of us already do it as a matter of habit. With a little thought, and perhaps a pencil and note pad, it should be fairly easy to organize what you already know about a patient into these contexts. Note, too, that we do not need to know everything about these contexts, only a few indicators that will help us understand the most salient facts about a patient's way of thinking and experience, as I will explain.

The object is not to know all the things listed here about every patient—which is quite impossible—but to have a systematic idea of the things that might be relevant for interpreting behavior and symptoms, and predicting responses to treatment plans.

When a problem arises in the therapeutic process, this model can be used to inventory what one already knows about a patient or patient group, and to think about what other information might be most useful in solving the problem, and where to get it.

In the *context of social class* falls information about how poor people are likely to be different from the middle and upper classes—the subject of this chapter. It is often necessary to further refine social class by ethnic group, such as Latino, Southeast Asian, or Native American, since poverty looks different according to its cultural variant. In this context, the questions to be answered are these:

- What do I know about this social class (and ethnic group) as a broad slice of American society that can help me understand the typical life experience of this patient?
- As a poor person what kinds of problems does he have; what resources are available or not available to him; how is he likely to view his health provider, his illness experience, and his treatment?
- What styles or subtypes are there within this group (for example, *villager* versus *warrior* identity), and which might this patient represent?

Most clients at a given health facility are living (however temporarily) in a geographically defined *service area*. In this context falls information about what the patient's neighborhood of residence is like, physically, economically, politically, and socially, as these things affect his experience. There may be several quite distinct types of neighborhoods in a service area, and it is important to know something about each of them, and how they differ. For example, certain streets might have high concentrations of a particular ethnic group or age group; or might be dominated by a particular institution like a factory, youth gang, drug cartel, or church. In this context, the questions to be answered are these:

- What do I know about this person's neighborhood that will help me to understand their experience and predict their behavior?
- What is the physical environment (style and quality of housing, hazards, climate, utilities, parks or greenery, traffic patterns)?
- What institutions and resources might be useful or harmful to him or her (churches, schools, government agencies, voluntary organizations, businesses, unions, sports teams, youth or criminal gangs, health care and public health, food and

pharmaceuticals outlets, police and fire, welfare, counseling, transportation, home help, entertainment)?

- What is the quality of each service, and who has access?
- What social characteristics might cause stress or provide help (racial and age composition and relationships, crime rates, police/community relations, church attendance, style of neighboring and friendship, kin networks, ethnic or class-based customs)?
- What and where are the constraints and opportunities of his or her economic situation (jobs, welfare, homelessness, charity activities, prices)?
- What linkages are there with outside resources and people (diocese, city hall, co-ethnics, union, veterans' organization)?

In the *context of gender*, we are not referring to the gender-specific biology of the disease or condition (which we hope we can assume is part of the professional's knowledge base), but to information about how the experience of being male or female affects the patient's experience of, and behavior toward, his or her health and illness. Questions to be answered in this context are these:

- What, in a given culture, are the social roles of males and females of the patient's age group (kind and amount of work done, relationships with spouse, children and other kin, access to nutrition, rest, health care, psychological support)?
- Given the occupation (including housewife or unemployed), how is gender likely to affect a person's work experience (rest, bathroom access, liquids and nutrition, social stresses involving co-workers, superiors or customers, exposure to hazards)?
- If the patient is a member of an at-risk group (homeless, mentally ill, handicapped, drug or alcohol abuser, HIV infected or chronically ill), how does this status interact with gender from a health standpoint (for example, exposure to sexual harassment in homeless shelters, and the like)?

In the *context of biography* falls information about how a particular life history and present circumstances interact with class and culture, neighborhood, and gender to produce a patient's unique understanding. This information will help explain the ori-

gin and nature of the health problem, and help in devising suggestions for action. Questions to be answered in this context are these:

- How are age, education, health status, and family status likely
  to affect the patient's problem?
- What experiences, knowledge, gifts, skills, personality traits,
  or handicaps might affect the illness or treatment?
- What is the patient's living situation like (quality and security
  of dwelling and surroundings, age/sex and relationship of
  household members, access/mobility problems, hazards,
  household demands, supports, and tensions)?
- Who is in the patient's network of relatives, friends, and acquaintances, and what is the frequency and nature of contact
  with each?
- What have been the important events in the patient's life lately
  (job loss or change, gain or loss of a close other, birth of a child,
  change of residence, arrest, new debt, religious experience)
  and how have they affected him or her?

Sources of Contextual Knowledge: Self, Patient, Neighborhood, Media

A moment ago, I said that we build up our picture of another person by mentally pasting together information that we have already
gleaned from many different sources, and that we continually add
to this picture as we browse for new knowledge in everyday life.
We can make this process a bit more efficient by looking at the
characteristics of the sources of our knowledge: What kind of information is located where? There is no logical or necessary sequence of sources that fits every information need, but let us
arbitrarily start with the most personal and immediate sources, and
go on to the more remote and impersonal ones.

The handiest source of information about a person or social
group is *oneself*:

- What do I already know objectively about the patient and the
  patient's class, culture, and community? (That is, what can I
  substantiate with relevant observation?)
- What stereotypes do I have about the patient or similar people

that I need to check against facts (the patient's values, lifestyle, abilities, feelings)?

- What feelings and attitudes do I have about people like the patient, where do these come from, and how do they affect our relationship? This can be especially useful in guarding against a certain false consciousness that often threatens relationships between social classes (see pages 78–85).

The second most intimate source of information is the *patient himself* and of course his immediate support group (especially those who accompany him to the clinic): What can I reasonably ask about his life—things that he and they will be conscious of, and not mind talking about?

- What is going on in their life right now?
- What is their experience and knowledge of his health and health problems?
- What, and whom, do they visualize as a potential help, and feel capable of making use of?
- What can they tell you about other possibly relevant features of their physical and social environment (location and access to help, nutrition, medicine, advice, financial support; sources of enjoyment, encouragement, or suffering; physical hazards)?
- What abilities do they have that might be tapped in treatment?

Moving to less personal sources, we come to the *neighborhood* as a direct source of information. A brief visual scrutiny of the neighborhood will reveal a great deal to the eye of an experienced health worker.

- What are the economic signs (banks versus check cashing businesses and pawn shops; well-kept housing versus subsidized projects and tenements; thriving commerce versus closed storefronts and idle people)?
- What are the class and cultural markers (dress, music, types of wares and services, languages)?
- What are the signs of anomie, disorganization, and chaos (graffiti, litter, vandalism, building security)?
- What are the signs of connectedness with the rest of the soci-

ety (transportation, libraries, parks, schools, churches, senior centers, cultural centers)?

Even more can be learned from talking casually with people in the streets and shops:

- What are the main problems of living or working here (safety, public services, price and availability of goods, housing, jobs, transportation, pollution)?
- What kinds of social distinctions do people make (race, gender, ethnicity, age, social class), and what are their attitudes toward each?
- What kinds of things bring people together (church, ethnic events, music, neighborhood projects, politics)?

The most general source of knowledge about patients is the *media*. By reading books, newspapers, magazines, and neighborhood newsletters; and by watching television and films, one can learn much about the class and ethnic context of health. This book, and those listed in the bibliography, are examples of media information on the poor:

- How do people in this group differ, in thinking and behavior, from people in other groups—especially the health worker's own?
- What has been the historical experience of this group, and how is that likely to affect thinking?
- What are some distinct subgroups or lifestyles of people in this group, and how does one recognize them?
- What are the popular images of this group in the mass media, and how accurate are they?
- What are the key economic and political issues for this group today?
- What are the key health and health care problems of this group?
- How are all these questions reflected in local and neighborhood news?

Table 3.1 gives a thumbnail summary of context levels and information sources for quick reference.

Table 3.1   *Levels and Sources of Information about Contexts*

	Media	Neighborhood	Patient	Self
Class/Culture	*Ethnography:* Differences from mainstream? History? Social types (how recognize)? *Popular Media:* Public images? Current issues?	Markers of class/culture (dress, food, language, institutions, etc.).	Markers of class/culture (dress, language, behaviors, attitudes).	Stereotypes of class/ culture, expectations, personal reactions.
Service Area	*Local news:* What issues? What groups? What resources?	*Physical:* Space, transport, safety, services, etc. *Social:* Groups, attitudes. *Economic:* Jobs, income, spending. *Political:* Action, belief.	Networks, neighborhood relations, access issues.	Own feelings and behavior in the neighborhood.
Gender	How is this person's gender an expression of cultural/ area norms?	What roles and attitudes do you see in relationships of the sexes? How different by age?	Personal experiences of gender and gender relations. Gender-specific ideas and expectations. Gender self-image.	Feelings and attitudes toward this gender, at this age, this ethnic group.
Biography	How is this life an expression of the class/cultural experience? What do I look for?	How does this environment shape personal experience?	Knowledge of, and attitudes toward, health, health care system, provider. Health history. Health related behavior.	Feelings and attitudes toward this person, as a person.

Other Sources of Knowledge: I. The Treatment Process

In chapter 1 I noted that healers and patients, being equally human, are in an important sense moral equals—that it is an act of hubris in a way for one person, however well trained, to take responsibility for another person's life or health. In a course I once took on medical ethics, the professor began by reminding us of this fact, and then asked us to consider, "For ethical purposes, what is a human being?" After we had struggled with this for half an hour, he asked us to consider the idea, "A human being is a being of finite freedom." We are free in the sense that our behavior is not strictly predetermined by our biology; but we are not infinitely free, because we are mortal. Certain behaviors are likely to lead to pain or death.

This freedom means that every human relationship is *reflexive* and *open ended*; whatever we do is based on our unique judgment and feelings at the time we do it, and cannot be predicted from the larger contexts of our culture, environment, or biography as a whole. Our shared contexts give us many common experiences, and greatly improve our ability to understand, to explain and influence, and to predict one another. But even if a health provider had detailed contextual information about every patient— which is impossible anyway—there would still be an element of psychosocial guesswork in every treatment.

Consequently, good practitioners routinely treat every health intervention as a psychosocial experiment—as a test of a set of hypotheses about the patient's social, psychological, and physical contexts. This means thinking of the outcome of a particular intervention as evidence—as data—that will be used to reexamine the original hypotheses. Although time demands nearly always limit the thoroughness of this process, ideally the provider:

(a) thinks about the psychosocial contexts (patient culture, experience, understanding, ability, environment) relevant to any particular intervention;

(b) seeks new contextual information if there does not seem to be enough;

(c) tries to design and present the intervention so that it is most likely to produce the desired results, given these contexts;

(d) tries to be fully aware of the relevant details (social ambiance of the interaction and who is present, exact vocabulary used, visual cues such as expression, posture, gesture, tone of voice) of interaction with the patient/ caretakers concerning the intervention;

(e) asks the patient/caretakers, if possible, to respond with feelings, problems, questions; and to feed back their understanding of instructions;

(f) adjusts the intervention in the light of any new information;

(g) records enough of these details so that they can be used to evaluate the psychosocial dimension of the outcome later;

(h) seeks information on the psychosocial features of the course and outcome of the problem (compliance problems, unexpected social/economic/environmental consequences) following the intervention;

(i) reviews this material as well as possible before further interventions;

(j) adjusts new interventions to fit the evidence of the psychosocial appropriateness of earlier ones.

Examples of the kinds of things one learns this way:

- Having a social worker or volunteer make transportation or child-care arrangements often improves the attendance of poor single mothers at appointments.
- If a chronically ill person will not take certain medications, it might be because they have experienced negative emotional or social results. (For example, incontinence resulting from diuretics). It may work to reduce the dose.
- Teaching an IV drug user how to inject in a more sterile way might spare him repeated abscesses and systemic infections.
- If depression is a complication of a poor patient's condition, it might help if the patient has an inexpensive way of participating actively in the treatment; for example, by growing and/ or preparing certain foods or herbs, by taking up a personally

meaningful activity (such as volunteer work) that requires exercise; or by teaching other patients how to deal with a similar problem.

■ Recognizing and responding to signs of anger in a patient may improve communication and build trust, thereby improving cooperation and outcome.

To the extent, then, that the provider is able to maintain contact with patients (which in fact might be virtually zero), one is in a good position to build up a fund of tested hypotheses about what kinds of patients, in a psychosocial sense, respond well to what kinds of interventions. I have seen this done, with great skill.

Other Sources of Knowledge: II. The Provider-Patient Relationship

Adjusting the treatment strategy to emerging knowledge about the context of the patient and the illness may help more in some cases than in others. As we all know, outcomes can be greatly affected by characteristics of the provider-patient relationship itself, somewhat independently of what goes on outside this relationship. Skill in recognizing one another's needs for knowledge, respect, and reassurance makes a great difference, as does the ability to share a language, communication style, and set of assumptions about how the relationship should be conducted.

Again, differences in social class between provider and patient sometimes contribute to difficulties in managing these features of the relationship. Here I will mention two common problems that health workers face in working with low-income clients: (1) overcompensation for class differences, and (2) denial or avoidance of the patient's anger and/or mistrust.

Overcompensation for Class Differences: The Dangers of 'Doing Good'

Health care settings where a large proportion of the clients are poor, such as inner city clinics and hospitals, emergency rooms, and community-based clinics, are often more stressful for the staff than other kinds of settings. For one thing, many (not all) low-income patients have multiple, complex health problems related, both as causes and as effects, to their economic situation. It is not uncommon to see in a single patient a combination of problems stemming from poor nutrition, poor housing or no housing at all, substance abuse, communicable disease, poor hygiene, medical neglect, and/or psychiatric illness.

Moreover, poor clients on average are for a variety of reasons more likely to miss appointments and to be noncompliant with prescribed regimen. A good clinician may have to spend more time negotiating the regimen with patients who have fewer resources and options, and more time explaining to patients with less knowledge. Then of course there is the problem of reimbursement. Health workers in these settings are generally paid less than those who treat a more affluent clientele.

All in all, health workers in settings most accessible to the poor often feel that they are caught in a dilemma. Visit for visit, their work is not as well paid as in other settings but at the same time their clients need more help, not less. Under the current reimbursement system, with its emphasis on provider productivity, this can be acutely frustrating.

Given this situation, there are often hidden psychological dangers in any desire to help others we consider less fortunate than ourselves—dangers to which even experienced health care providers are vulnerable. These dangers arise from two syndromes that usually go together:

- an unrecognized desire to be admired and rewarded for one's attitude of self-sacrifice,
- a romanticization of the poor motivated by (a) the sense that the health worker and his/her clients are equally oppressed, or (b) a guilty sense that one is not doing enough for one's clients. (Oddly enough, it is possible to find both these perceptions in the same person.)

The first problem can lead us to expect more emotional support and understanding from clients, co-workers, and superiors than we are likely to get in our work with the poor. Feeling chronically undervalued, some of us are inclined to interpret criticism, or sometimes even a lack of enthusiastic support, as a lack of due recognition for our moral excellence. At its worst, this can result in a loss of insight into one's own performance, and from there to a deterioration in that performance and in relationships with clients and other workers.

The remedy for this is to be as aware as possible of our actual motives in working with the poor, and as open as possible to the opinions of others about our performance. There is a difference between demanding respect and appreciation for good work, and expecting to be loved for the warmth of our hearts regardless of performance. Everyone occasionally loses sight of this difference, but if we feel constantly victimized in our job, this might be at least part of the problem.

The second problem usually goes with the first. Both over-identification and guilt concerning the condition of the poor can lead to failure to recognize one's anger toward clients, and failure to identify client behaviors that need to be changed. Poor patients, like any other sick people, can be demanding, irritable, withdrawn, stubbornly noncompliant, manipulative, and ungrateful. It is quite natural for the health worker to dislike these behaviors, and even occasionally to build up resentment toward the worst offenders. Ordinarily, such feelings can be resolved with the patient directly and honestly; but not where guilt is involved.

Our own unidentified anger is a threat to our self-image as caregivers, and hiding this anger from ourselves becomes a major project. It is often a symptom of this project that we are unable to confront a poor patient about unacceptable behavior, or to challenge their truthfulness. Our intellectual justification of this inability is often a romanticized view of poor clients—a view that portrays their villainy either as something else, or as something excusable. We forget that some poor people are well aware of this tendency, and have long since learned how to make the most of it.

In addition to the suffering this causes us as health workers, it creates problems for others. The patient's behavior may be leading in a self-destructive direction, yet it goes unchallenged. Manipulative patients may be absorbing resources (especially time) that are needed by other patients and colleagues. Our suffering is likely to aggravate our feelings of victimization, our demands for attention, and our hypersensitivity to criticism. In the worst cases, we may take the side of a manipulative patient against others, which wreaks havoc with important work relationships.

The remedy for this problem is

- to be aware and accepting of our negative feelings toward clients;
- to learn to distinguish carefully between acceptable and unacceptable behavior, and confront the latter no matter whose it is;
- to be suspicious of any portrayal of the poor as morally better than other people.

I have noticed that health workers who themselves come from poor backgrounds are often relatively free of these problems (although they may well have other ones). I am tempted to say that many formerly poor health professionals seem to work with the poor mainly because they feel comfortable working with the poor, and not because they see what they do as a form of self-sacrifice or a way of expiating their sins. I have often found myself studying such people as role models and seeking advice from them.

Denial or Avoidance of the Patient's Anger or Mistrust

A colleague of mine is the director of a midwifery unit in a large urban hospital that serves many low-income clients. The midwives are proud of the high standards of care on their unit.

One evening a Latin American patient who had been seen throughout the thirty-eight weeks of her pregnancy came in to the clinic and said, "There is something wrong with my baby. I know there is. I have to have it now, or something terrible is going to happen. I want a cesarean right now." She was immediately thoroughly examined, but no danger signs were detected. The fetal heartbeat was normal, the baby was moving, the mother had no fever or other evident symptoms. There was no dilation or contractions.

Compromising with her wishes, the staff tried unsuccessfully to induce labor over the next day and a half. But having been trained to value childbirth as a natural function, and still not seeing signs of danger, they finally sent the woman home at seven in the evening on the second day, telling her to call immediately if anything happened. Until the moment she left, the patient argued that she knew she was right, and that they should give her a cesarean.

At five the next morning, her husband called, saying her water had broken, and asking for a pain prescription. He was told to bring her to the unit immediately. However, two hours later, the husband appeared at the unit without the patient, asking again for pain medication. When he was finally convinced to bring her in, she was found to have a uterine infection, and the baby was dead. Later she cursed the midwives, saying that they had ignored her out of racial prejudice.

Six months later, some of the midwives were still in psychotherapy, attempting to heal the emotional trauma of this case.

Our ideal of the healing encounter is one in which a blameless and grateful supplicant places her trust in a competent health worker, in search of a mutual alliance to secure a healthy outcome. But regardless of social class or income, Americans today tend to believe they have a right to care that is humane and highly effective. Add to such expectations the heightened sensitivity and weakened emotional resources of a sick person. Blend into the mix the relatively slow, inaccurate, impersonal, and confusing health care bureaucracy that all but the wealthiest patients confront. Multiply this by the number of times a low-income person is likely to have encountered inhumane and insulting conditions in her search for care (discussed in chapter 6). Then calculate the likelihood that any given healing encounter involves an angry and mistrustful person—if not the patient, her relatives—regardless of the actual behavior of the provider at the time.

When confronted with anger or mistrust that we do not share, the natural tendency of most of us is either to deflect it by showing sympathy, or simply to get away from it as quickly as possible. If the negative feelings are openly directed at us, and we cannot easily withdraw, many of us (myself included) tend to become defensive and dismiss them as irrational and irrelevant. If such feelings are expressed more subtly, we have a tendency to hope they will simply go away if we ignore them.

What we should do, of course, is explore patient anger and mistrust directly; but this is difficult to do even when we know the patient's personality and culture well, and feel reasonably secure in such an exchange. When we feel unsure about our ability to communicate, and do not know what to expect, it is a fearsome task indeed.

And there is to be sure a huge variety of situations in which patient anger and mistrust are found. The history of the patient's encounters with health providers and other authorities, the way his culture shapes the perception of relationships and the handling of emotions, the actual situation in which the encounter happens, and the patient's unique personality and immediate mental status—all contribute to the complexity of the situation. But as the case I just gave illustrates, the effects of untreated anger can be truly devastating.

For those who have not had thorough training in dealing with angry or suspicious clients, I recommend these steps:

1. Try to be *self-conscious about your own habits* of dealing with this problem. How do you recognize it? What characteristics of the angry/mistrustful person or persons (age, sex, race, ethnicity, social class, state of health, etc.) affect your response, and how? What characteristics of the situation (setting, presence of others, roles, time of day, etc.) make a difference? What are your feelings (anxiety, guilt, and defensiveness are normal) and actions (ignoring, withdrawing, intellectualizing, blaming others, arguing, listening and facilitating discussion)?

2. *Examine the situations* in which you frequently encounter anger/mistrust in your work. (If there aren't any, why?) Who is angry/suspicious, when, and why?

3. *Discuss with others* in your milieu how they deal with anger/mistrust, *and observe* them. Do some people have skills and attitudes that complement yours?

4. If you feel that you could and should improve your ability to deal with anger or suspicion, try to *arrange for professional training* to that end. Get a *professional consultation* on possible changes in your own procedures or those of your workplace that could make things easier.

Exercises and Study Questions

1. *Rate yourself* on your awareness of the various contexts of your patients' health. For any given patient:

   - Can you point to his or her neighborhood on a map? Have you ever been to that neighborhood? Have you ever been to the patient's house, or driven by it?
   - How long has the patient lived there? Where did he/she come from? How many places has he/she lived in the last few years?
   - What is the patient's ethnicity and religion? How important are these factors to the patient? What do you know about that ethnicity or religion?
   - What are the patient's important relationships? Have you met any of these people, or do you know anything about them?
   - What is the patient's work, and where? Have you ever been to the place, or to one like it? What kind of environment is it?

2. Make up a *one-page face sheet* that allows you to fill in the basic contextual data on all your patients. Organize it in a way that makes the most sense to you. Try using it to (1) find out how much you know/don't know about each patient that might be useful, (2) get more information, (3) improve your effectiveness.

PART II

Poverty Under the Microscope

CHAPTER 4

Why Does It Exist?

In Utopia, there would be no poverty. That is one thing the affluent and the poor can agree on. There is also general agreement that society has an obligation to reduce as far as possible the suffering due to poverty, and ideally, to eliminate it altogether. Many reforms and many revolutions have taken root in this principle. Accordingly, social philosophy and science have for centuries studied and debated the causes and remedies of poverty, and there is very little new that can be said about the subject. In this chapter I will discuss the leading explanations and beliefs about who the poor are and what accounts for their sociological and demographic reality.

It is important for health professionals to be familiar with these ideas. As we will see in later chapters, ideas about how to approach the health of the poor are closely tied to ideas about the causes and cures of their economic situation. For example, the policy of removing low-income people from the welfare roles (now proceeding on a large scale) is based on the theory that welfare payments handicap recipients by reducing their motivation to work. But the effects of such a policy on health will depend on the ability of the poor to get adequate housing, nutrition, and care by other means; and this in turn will depend on their whole relation to the broader economy and society.

To know where a clinic's clientele fits in the economic geography is to be able to think realistically about patients' options for care, and this in turn can translate into better understanding of how services can be designed to better meet their needs. For example, my town is currently in a health care crisis, since cuts to the government subsidies of clinics serving the poor have made it impossible to handle the health needs of the uninsured—those with neither private nor public (Medicare, Medicaid, indigent care) coverage. In trying to develop a plan to deliver primary care services to this population, one needs to know not only who they are demographically, but also what is happening economically to the area, and consequently to them.

Most important of all, in my view, personal relationships between providers and poor clients also can benefit from a broad social perspective on poverty. Patient and provider are drawn infinitely closer when they see themselves together as actors in an historical drama—transformed from mutual enigma to co-participants in a familiar story. Our mutual individuality becomes so much clearer to us.

The Dynamics of Poverty

In the first chapter, we defined poverty not as a simple economic condition, but as a state of demoralization, where people lack all or most of the minimum ingredients we accept as the basis of a decent life, including hope, safety and security, respect, and mental and physical health. We mentioned the difficulty of knowing, based on simple statistics like income, who is really poor and who is not. In moving to the discussion of poverty at the macro level, I have no simple solution to this difficulty, and most of the ideas I will talk about are based on studies of such indirect measures as income and living costs, education, employment, and morbidity. However, many of my sources, such as Michael Katz, Janet Fitchen, David Snow and Leon Anderson, Philippe Bourgois, and Jonathan Kozol, also have thorough ethnographic knowledge of poor communities that I think keep them from seriously misinterpreting the macroeconomic data.

Neither can one really speak about the pathways to poverty in a general way, since there are various distinct dynamics. Small town versus inner city, age, employment, health, and race tend to divide the processes and experiences of impoverishment into types. There are always individual poor families that do not fit into any of these types as well. Observers who are determined to see poverty as a self-inflicted condition brought on by lack of determination, or good sense, or moral backbone will always be able to cite anecdotes to support their view, because in truth there are many such people. There are also those who choose poverty over a respectability that feels to them, for private reasons, humiliating.

In this chapter, I will focus on what I see as the causes of poverty for those whom I think are the great majority—not the neurotically proud or self-pitying, or the cognitively impaired. I will try to sketch the major current social and economic factors in American society that have the effect of increasing inequality, and making it difficult for the majority of the poor—those who want to earn a decent life—to change their circumstances. The factors I will discuss are the decline of jobs in manufacturing, the mobility of capital, suburbanization, racial segregation, and the politics of inequality. Most poor families find themselves the victims of several of these factors, which interact in complex ways. Taken as a whole, the forces in question add up to a process I call the *verticalization of society*: an increasingly wealthy, powerful, and self-serving minority, and an increasingly poor, powerless, and isolated working class.

The Decline of Manufacturing Jobs and the Mobility of Capital

American prosperity until the 1960s was driven primarily by growth in manufacturing jobs. Then several things began to change. One was the increasing replacement of human power by machinery, a process that accelerated greatly when electronics came in, thanks to inventions like the transistor. Another was the sudden and dramatic development of manufacturing capacity abroad, in countries where relatively low wages kept the prices of products low. This expansion was, in turn, made possible by the accumulation of capital in the industrial countries, now available for investment overseas (Frobel et al. 1977). Coupled with these trends, communication and transportation technology sharply improved, making it much easier to do business over long distances and resulting in the decentralization of manufacturing operations.

Before the Second World War, manufacturers tended to base efficiency on large-scale operations, located close to equally centralized sources of fuel, transportation, labor, and raw materials. In the low-income neighborhoods that clustered around these manufacturing and trade centers, workers with few skills could often find low-paid but fairly steady work. As I mentioned in chapter 2, factory work tended to be well suited to the social and psychological needs of poor men. In the factory, men were often poorly paid and subject to serious dangers, but it was a type of work where they could demonstrate valued qualities—strength, endurance, courage, quickness—to peers who shared their values and understood their customs. Moreover, if a man could keep his health and stay out of trouble, he could often advance modestly in pay and job security. With the increasing productivity of the economy, most workers could count on small increases in real wages over time. Such poverty, as Katz says, "existed within a context of hope" (1995, 78).

When automation, cheap imports, and *outsourcing* (contracting abroad for finished components) began to erode manufacturing jobs, higher profits and improvements in communications and transportation also allowed manufacturing to move operations easily. Factories relocated in areas—both domestic and abroad—where wages and taxes were low, regulations and unions weak.

Today, those "rust belt" poor who have enough education and social skills may find jobs in an expanding service sector—hotels and restaurants, office services, transportation, data processing, and so on. However, under the new conditions, many poor residents of inner cities cannot make a living wage. They do not have the education for skilled office work, and even most low-paid, unskilled service jobs require men to work in social situations that are unfamiliar and extremely difficult for them. Bourgois shows graphically, in his study of working-class Puerto Ricans in New York, how discouraging it is for these men. Accustomed to a hypermasculine culture where tolerating disrespect could mean social—and even literal—death, some find themselves in menial office jobs where they are expected to accept (smilingly!) contemptuous treatment from young female supervisors. This is something that would not happen on a factory floor. Many men prefer work in the informal economy—doing "bootleg" construction or repair work, unlicensed buying and selling, or dealing drugs—where they work among people like themselves, and (like the factory worker) turn their toughness to advantage (Bourgois 1995, 143–173).

Unemployment—and employment in the informal economy—are then major effects of the decline of manufacturing; but they are probably not the greatest poverty-producing effects. Other major effects are underemployment and low wages in the formal economy. America's sixty million families whose income fall below 150 percent of the official federal poverty line usually cannot afford basic necessities like food, shelter, clothes, fuel, and education (Schwarz and Volgy 1993). The heads of about half of these families work year round—either full-time or part-time—and about another fourth work more than twenty-six weeks per year. Their poverty results from the fact that they do not work enough, and/ or do not get paid enough, to live decently.

The reasons for this situation are of course complex. A permanent shortage of jobs assures that there are always plenty of people willing to work for less than a living wage, and that fired or laid-off, low-skilled employees can always be replaced quickly. Accordingly, employment in this country has come to be structured around these features of the work force. In fact, for many years it has been an open policy of the government to keep unemployment high in order to keep inflation in check (Schiller 1984).

In chapter 5, we will discuss the currently popular argument that welfare costs would be reduced if current recipients were required to work. The underlying notion, that there are abundant jobs waiting for these people, is simply not true. Studies of job availability in selected cities have shown that the number of appropriate jobs in large U.S. cities is usually a small fraction of the number of people out of work. One study in New York found that there were 5,000 standing jobs available, but 139,000 *officially* unemployed (that is, listed with employment agencies) and over 200,000 heads of households on welfare (Bernstein 1970, 6). The New York study did not examine the qualifications needed for these jobs, or whether poor people might reasonably apply for most of them. A study in Washington D.C. did so, with discouraging results:

> At the time of the study, 36,400 people were counted as "unemployed," and 28,000 adults were receiving welfare payments. Yet 3,038 jobs were listed in the paper. . . . Closer examination of the ads revealed . . . [that] most of the jobs required educational attainments or experience that the poor simply do not have. In all, only 354 of the job vacancies—12 percent—were jobs that poor people might get. Phone calls to the employers listing these jobs confirmed that nearly all the job vacancies were filled, usually in a day or two. (Schiller 1974, 53).

Let us assume that there were twice as many appropriate jobs available but unlisted, and that the unemployed would be able to find these unlisted jobs. The chances of getting work would still have been roughly three in one hundred.

Yet another study, in Austin, Texas, compared the job experience of homeless people with the requirements of the 2,371 jobs listed in the newspaper, and found that there was a possible match in 112 of these jobs—4.7 percent. The authors comment, "This mismatch becomes even more striking when we consider that the majority of the remaining jobs for which the homeless might qualify under ideal conditions are unavailable to them because they lack such requisite job resources as references, drivers' licenses, tools, clean clothes, a telephone number, and a permanent address" (Snow and Anderson 1993, 117). The federal government itself has estimated the cost of job creation and job training needed to move just one segment of the welfare caseload—AFDC mothers—into jobs. The figure is $15 billion, a project that would, in DeParle's words, "rival the Works Projects Administration, which employed 3.3 million people at the height of the Depression" (DeParle 1994, 48). In 1999, three years after Congress cut welfare, the Clinton administration announced that they are requesting from Congress $15 billion in investment funds over five years to reduce poverty. From the point of view of the poor family, what this all means is that jobs currently are not only hard to find, they don't pay well enough to make ends meet, and they are easily lost—due to cost-cutting measures, the inability of the worker to meet demands, or the relocation of the job somewhere else. Many poor people have to move from job to job, rarely gaining enough seniority or experience to attain security or decent pay.

The Suburbanization of the Countryside

Another complex of factors, this time having to do with the geography of housing, transportation, and retail marketing, has produced a physical segregation of the affluent and the poor that greatly restricts the upward mobility of the latter. As a shorthand, I call this the suburbanization of the countryside, since that is something familiar to most of us. The main dynamics driving suburbanization are the desire of the middle class for home ownership, and for a child-friendly environment with open space and good schools; the concentration of agriculture in the hands of large, industrialized producers, which renders marginal agricultural land unprofitable; the desire of the real estate industry (banks and other land and title speculators, building contractors, building materials producers, realtors, and real estate law firms) for continuous profits; the participation of the retail trade and transportation industries in the housing profit scramble; the influence of these powerful industries on state and local government policies with respect to housing, schools, transportation, and taxes.

The process can be visualized as a set of trends which does not follow a linear sequence, but rather is interlocking and mutually reinforcing: low real estate prices in rural areas near cities; growth of housing affordable for middle-class commuters in these areas; improvement of roads and utilities connecting these areas with cities; rising real estate values as amenities improve; relocation of more and more middle-income urban families to these areas, leaving inner city neighborhoods with declining average incomes; decline of retail trades in said neighborhoods; decline of inner city tax base, both residential and commercial; decline of city services (schools, libraries, parks, police and fire protection, street and building maintenance, refuse collection) due to lower tax base; shift of economic growth either to urban centers accessible to suburbanites, or to the suburbs themselves, lowering job prospects in city neighborhoods; discriminatory government and business policies with respect to these ghettoized urban neighborhoods (location of toxic hazards and polluting industries; red lining against credit; relocation of essential shops and services elsewhere, etc.); large scale destruction of cheap housing in these communities, to make way for freeways, restricted (subsidized) government housing, or more profitable commercial uses; high concentrations of discriminated minorities, and of "problem" families and individuals in the subsidized housing neighborhoods.

A parallel but related process also produces pockets of hard core poverty in rural areas farther from the cities: decline of small-scale agriculture on marginal land leads to falling population and land values; businesses and government services in small towns disappear or are consolidated in suburban centers; low housing costs in depleted small towns attract low-income families; deteriorating conditions of housing, services, and infrastructure affects appearance and reputation of neighborhoods; class segregation accelerates as more affluent families move out.

These are not, of course, the only processes that produce, or deepen, poverty. Many small towns that have always been poor have been adversely affected by rural industrialization, under which mines either lay off workers and bring in machinery, or are depleted rapidly; while meanwhile large-scale mechanized farming and transportation puts small farmers out of business (Fitchen 1981; Couto 1982, ch. 3). These processes are related to urban industrialization in various ways also, and result in problems similar to those of declining urban neighborhoods—the downward spiral of isolation, loss of resources, and powerlessness.

One way of visualizing the effects of these trends on poverty is to think of them as a kind of sorting process, whereby people who have relatively few resources and skills tend to collect in areas where living is cheap, while those whose resources allow them a choice of living environments tend to congregate in areas where

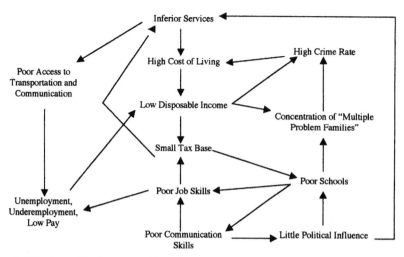

FIGURE 4.1. The Downward Spiral

living is more expensive. In the latter, of course, there are better government services, more open space, and less visible evidence of misery. This sorting process sets in motion two spirals. Those families who find themselves surrounded by good schools, well-educated (and perhaps influential) neighbors, good jobs, and good infrastructure, and possessed of the clothes, cars, skills, and cash to take full advantage of these things, find themselves using these advantages to climb, with a little luck, an upward spiral toward greater affluence. A downward spiral catches those who find themselves in overcrowded, substandard housing and schools, surrounded by the underemployed and the illegally employed, remote from good jobs and services, discriminated against by the affluent world, and lacking a chance to acquire the skills needed to interact with the upward-spiral people.

The cumulative, or spiral, effect of the two positions can be better understood, perhaps, if we offer a diagram of some of the interactions between features of each one (figure 4.1).

Racial Segregation

Although as I mentioned in chapter 1, over 60 percent of America's poor are white, no close observer can fail to notice that the inner city communities with the highest concentrations of poverty are overwhelmingly nonwhite. Kozol writes,

> A demographic forecast by the city's planning agency predicts that the population of the Bronx—both North and South—half of which was white in 1970, and nearly a quarter of which was white in 1990, will be entirely black and Hispanic by the early years of the next century, outside of a handful of de facto segregated enclaves of white people and a few essentially detached communities like parts of Riverdale. By that time, the Bronx and Harlem and Washington Heights will make up a vast and virtually uninterrupted ghetto with a population close to that of Houston, Texas, which is America's fourth-largest city. (1995, 192)

Of the forty-eight thousand people living in the blighted public housing tract of Mott Haven, which Kozol observed closely, 1.7 percent were white. Bourgois reports that East Harlem—where the poverty rate is 40 percent and 48 percent of males over sixteen are unemployed—is 52 percent Puerto Rican and 39 percent black (1995, 7).

For the country as a whole, about 31 percent of blacks and 29 percent of Hispanics are officially poor, as compared with 11 percent of whites (Katz 1989, 241). Elsewhere Katz notes,

> Although the proportion of African Americans who are poor has declined steeply since the 1960s, the proportion who are chronically without jobs has risen sharply. As a result, the chronically jobless compose an ever larger share of the poor, and African Americans constitute a greater share of those chronically without jobs now than in earlier periods. This connection between race, urban poverty, and dissociation from the labor market is new in American history. (1995, 79)

Katz also notes "In the 1980s . . . wage inequality between black and white men increased at all educational levels," due to the failure of education in predominantly black neighborhoods to prepare students for modern workforce participation (1995, 79).

What accounts for the increasing segregation of poor people of color? I believe the answer is complex, but demonstrates a subtle and pervasive American elitism that is both racial and class based. This elitism is the result of the we/they reflex, which judges poorer or less educated people as unworthy of compassion or trust, and makes the unreflective assumption that people of color are (until proven otherwise) poorer or less educated than whites. This reflex finds expression in housing, employment and promotion, and the quality of services of all kinds.

As an activist in my own community, I have seen basically decent middle-class whites react with surprising hostility to proposals that would move toward residential desegregation of class and race. They do not use racist or classist arguments. They talk about the inconvenience and risk that would be imposed on their neighborhoods if even a few units of high density housing were located there. They consider that the poor of any color are better off in neighborhoods "where people know and help each other," (which, in truth, few people do on most affluent blocks). Not being students of social history, they fail to see their actions as details of the bigger picture which they themselves deplore.

In employment, the shift from a manufacturing to a service economy has meant that more and more jobs put low-income workers in direct contact with more educated clients and supervisors. Both real and imagined cultural differences between these workers—especially if they are African or Latino Americans—and middle-class Euro-Americans make management-worker relations difficult. Employers fear that greater adjustments will have to be made in interpersonal attitudes if one hires nonwhites, and that making these adjustments will lower efficiency. Over and over one hears the complaint from middle-class executives (of all colors) that such-and-such nonwhite employee "just doesn't fit in" to the workplace culture. Color is very often seen as the overriding factor, and subsequently used to evaluate new job candidates.

Racial discrimination in the quality of services people receive in predominantly white settings puts pressure on nonwhite families to seek services from people of their own color, and thereby to gravitate to communities where such services are available. It is commonly said, for example, that nonwhite Americans "underuse" racially and class-integrated services such as nursing homes, health fairs, and clinics.

Notice how all these processes are self-perpetuating in nature—they are reciprocal, circular, and interlocking. The geographic isolation of the affluent and the poor erodes everyone's comfort and skill in interclass and interracial encounters. This discomfort lowers everyone's chance of experience in integrated living and work settings, and makes it harder to build such settings. Earlier, I spoke of the segregation of the poor as a sorting process, whereby the casualties in our competitive society are gradually stripped of the means to reverse their downward spiral. Using this metaphor, race is an added increment of disadvantage, increasing the odds that a family will find itself in the downward spiral, and be required to join a community where this spiral is the norm. This process, plus the discomfort of the races with integrated settings, results in the concentration of nonwhites in more and more isolated urban ghettos.

The Role of Political Culture

Since poverty has always been a matter of concern to society, to explain its persistence we must examine why the machinery of collective action consistently fails to alleviate it. In the next chapter I will look more closely at welfare politics, but here I want to consider the cultural context in which the political treatment of the poor takes place.

I began this book by referring to the distinction between the deserving and the undeserving poor—those who are clearly physically or situationally unable to care for themselves, and those who are judged capable of doing so by society. The deserving poor generally include the elderly, children, and the sick and disabled. Many observers of poverty have pointed out that the national governments of the wealthier modern societies do try to relieve their suffering by providing them with at least minimum support: housing, medical care, food, and other necessities. In the United States we have Social Security and Medicare for the old and disabled, and Temporary Assistance to Needy Families (TANF)—formerly called Aid to Families of Dependent Children (AFDC)—for children, and so on.

With respect to the undeserving poor, however, most national governments in capitalist countries take a different role—that of preserving the peace and well-being of the society at large, by preserving the lives of the destitute, and preventing them from rioting (Simmel 1908; Piven and Cloward 1971). The most vigorous efforts to relieve general poverty in the United States, for example, took place during periods of widespread and often violent public protest—the Great Depression of the 1930s, and the Civil Rights Movement of the 1960s. Two facts are noteworthy about both these periods. First, in both eras the security of the nonpoor was widely felt to be at risk. Second, social perceptions of the causes of poverty shifted, partially erasing the deserving/undeserving distinction. Millions of able-bodied poor were temporarily freed from blame, in the first instance because of widespread economic crisis, and in the second instance due to a new awareness of racial discrimination.

In any case, contrary to prevailing political rhetoric, the exercise of conscience with regard to the undeserving poor—meaning attempts to relieve their suffering on humanitarian grounds—usually has been left to private charity and local government. This has several important effects on the persistence of poverty. First, it enormously complicates collective response to poverty, by impeding consistent policies, and by leaving the issue a matter of power struggle among local constituencies. Second, as we have seen in the case of inner city ghettos, it allows sharp local economic inequalities to dictate equally sharp—and self-enlarging—inequalities of lifestyle and hope.

Most importantly, the parochialization of poverty maximizes distance between the poor and their advocates on one hand, and the loci of real political power on the other hand. Legions of real political issues facing actual poor families or communities can be used as examples of how this perpetuates their condition. I live in one of the most politically liberal counties in America, with a high rate of poverty (20 percent below federal guideline). Yet local efforts to improve housing, health care, or education are consistently frustrated by policies or decisions made farther up the power hierarchy. For example:

1. California law forbids not only the raising of local property tax valuations in keeping with rising real estate values under any circumstances, but also the adoption of other local taxes without a two-thirds vote of the electorate. The resulting limit on taxes helps property owners send their children to private schools, while public education suffers from a shrunken budget, even when there is majority support for more local taxes.

2. Recent cuts in state and federal subsidies for health care have resulted in dangerous losses to the budgets of local clinics that serve the poor. To stay solvent, these clinics have had to stop taking uninsured low-income patients—a result the city government is trying to rectify by coordinating volunteer health providers.

3. The state health department retroactively rescinded its negotiated Medicaid rate at one of the local clinics, and threatened to collect several hundred thousand dollars in back overpayments covering three years. The clinic remains open only thanks to its strong local support. Should it close, most of its 17,000 annual patient visits would have to be absorbed by nearby emergency rooms, which are already overcrowded.

Let us look at the problems, then, that confront efforts of the poor to organize for political change. One is their geographic and social isolation from mainstream society. Individual neighborhoods do frequently come together to work for change on a small scale, such as the removal of crack houses or corrupt local officials. However, such neighborhoods are (a) largely isolated from those with money, education, and access to power and communications; (b) often fragmented by cultural divisions; (c) plagued by internal instability as people change or lose jobs, support systems, or residences; (d) sensitive to threats of retaliation by landlords, employers, rival factions, or city officials.

Another major barrier to effective political action among the poor is one that community organizers often experience but rarely talk about: Any voluntary cooperative group has to delegate some authority and share some resources in order to get work done. In urban neighborhoods with little history of cooperation and the knowledge and trust that go with it, there is great uncertainty about leadership. When the members of a group have very few personal resources to start with, even small amounts of money, power, or prestige easily become subjects of destructive personal competition within the group. I have seen many cooperative efforts founder over seemingly small matters that evoked jealousy and mistrust among potential leaders—especially the management of money and the delegation of authority. I will return to these points in chapter 8, when we discuss community organizing.

These barriers to the development of power on the part of the poor, formidable though they are, do not explain one of the most troubling political problems: Many observers have noted that voting rates among the poor tend to be much lower than among other economic groups, due to an overwhelming pessimism about politics (Howell 1973; Fitchen 1981; Kozol 1995). I do not believe there is any simple explanation for this, but it can be partly understood if we think about typical experiences of life among the poor versus the nonpoor.

Most people with plentiful resources are accustomed to making and carrying out complex, long term plans—plans that have major effects on their lives, and that bear at least some fruit more often than not. If things do not go well at first, or if unforeseen problems arise, such people often have the reserves to persevere, to cope, or try other strategies, without giving up their goals. In other words, they are accustomed to visualizing the future carefully and planfully, to having their plans considered seriously by others, and to feeling effective when their plans bear fruit.

Such people have access to the material means (savings, collateral, reliable income, tools, transportation, telecommunications, purchasing power) and the skills (advanced literacy, experience with institutions and authority) to carry out their plans. By their dress, grooming, speech and confident demeanor, they generally look successful, and are taken seriously in their transactions. Most importantly, they feel connected to the institutions of their society, in a deeply personal way. These institutions are run by, and for, people like themselves, according to goals and strategies that are not fundamentally different from their own.

In this context, political participation makes sense. Planned actions whose outcome is uncertain, and whose results may be many months or even years in coming are part of one's regular repertoire. One is accustomed to visualizing the positive effects of one's actions. Others are expected to take one's opinions seriously, and to behave, on the whole, according to a logic that is transparent.

As we discussed in the last chapter, the experience of poor people is usually quite different. Where basic needs like income, housing, and transportation are highly insecure, the chance of failure at any new venture increases dramatically as a function of time. Operating close to the margin of one's resources means that even a small setback can completely destroy the plan. Securing help and encouragement from others is extremely difficult when one is perceived as overwhelmingly needy, or unlikely to succeed. Accordingly, life takes on the existential quality we spoke of in chapter 2. Plans are kept short-term, and are often dropped or switched to take advantage of immediate opportunities or cope with immediate threats. Time spent visualizing the future and tinkering with its possibilities is likely to produce discouragement and depression. Such activities do not become a habit.

Moreover, one is accustomed to being ignored by mainstream people and institutions. To preserve self-respect, one has to accept one's marginality somehow. As I have said, pride tends to be based on one's ability to endure disappointment and hardship, rather than on one's ability to change it or escape from it. Kozol quotes a minister of a South Bronx church: "People protest specific actions of the city. They protested the waste burner. But there's a sense of powerlessness that makes it hard to keep up a momentum. The reality of the streets is a continuing reminder and compelling reenactment of despair" (1995, 81).

In this context, political participation may seem to make little sense. Even the most liberal political figures seem to represent a set of institutions and a way of life on which one has turned one's back. To put energy into a long-term process, like orderly political change, is equally alien. And to believe that a better future may be within one's reach is often to weaken one of the most powerful elements of one's self-respect—pride in toughness.

This look at the big picture of the political and economic context of poverty in contemporary America is, I admit, enough to discourage anyone. But there is another side to the picture: Poor communities can and do change their conditions. In later chapters we will discuss some examples of successful change, and look at the conditions that seem to make such change possible. First, though, we must confront more closely those features of this unlovely picture that most closely affect health and health care: The current politics of health and welfare, and the health conditions of the poor.

Exercises and Study Questions

1. What explanations of poverty are offered in the mainstream news media? How much space is devoted to such explanations?

2. What is meant by the word *individualism*? Discuss how the economics of poverty are related to individualism. (Are Swedes less individualistic than Americans?)

3. What economic policies might reduce inequality in the United States? Where might effective support for such policies be found?

4. State the basic principles of capitalism and socialism. Are there alternative economic theories?

5. Design a project for educating people in your community about the causes of local economic inequality. Who would your audience be? How would you reach them? What materials and teaching methods would you use? How would you evaluate the results?

The Poor on the Picture Tube

CHAPTER 5

The "Debates" on Welfare and Health Care Reform

A decent provision for the poor is the true test of civilization.
                                —Samuel Johnson (d.1784)

The function of the state as the guardian of the public well-being assures that the question of what to do about poverty will always be a concern of politics. Poverty poses a threat, not just to its direct victims, but—as a source of strife and discontent, disease, vice and crime, environmental harm, and public cost—to the affluent as well. As nations pass through social and economic change, periods of upheaval tend to alternate with periods of stability. Accordingly, people feel less secure about their future during certain epochs. Their ideas about what causes poverty, what threats it poses, and what ought to be done about it are affected, and these changes are reflected in political policy and law. I mentioned in the last chapter how the Great Depression and the Civil Rights Movement temporarily changed American ideas on the issue, and left their legacy of welfare and civil rights legislation.

The chief legacy of the Depression was of course the Social

Security Act of 1935, which established government benefits for the elderly, the blind and the disabled (OASDI), and for widowed and abandoned mothers and their children (ADC, later called AFDC). With the exception of the working-class elderly and the disabled, the effect of this legislation on chronic poverty was not very great at first. For the first twenty years or so, both the number of women eligible for AFDC and the percentage who participated (about one-quarter) was relatively small, yielding 2.2 million recipients in 1955. These numbers began to change dramatically in the late 1950s, as new social attitudes began to produce higher divorce rates and more open acceptance of unwed pregnancy, and the welfare changes of the 1960s accelerated this change.

The legacy of the Kennedy-Johnson War on Poverty of the 1960s is more complicated. Having fought a very large war quite successfully and having entered a period of unparalleled prosperity, the country was feeling confident about solving its social problems by means of a similar mass mobilization. The belief became widespread in government that programs linking welfare with job training and improved opportunities would eventually eliminate poverty as a public burden, much as World War II had helped to eliminate the jobs programs of the 1930s.

Accordingly, federal welfare payments were raised substantially, eligibility was expanded, and those eligible were encouraged to participate. Job training programs were encouraged, and the individual states developed a number of plans. In 1967 the "thirty plus a third" rule was added to federal welfare provisions, allowing beneficiaries to keep the first $30 of earned income, plus a third of anything above that, up to a limit of allowable income, without losing their welfare benefits.

However, moving welfare recipients to jobs turned out to be much more difficult that predicted—partly because there was never any coordination between welfare and labor-market policy. One result of all this was a dramatic decrease in poverty among some sectors; but another result was an explosion in the number of recipients of AFDC, and its cost. By 1972 there were over ten million AFDC recipients (Smolensky et al. 1995). Although their cost to the government was still small relative to other programs (2.5 percent of the federal budget), this growth set the stage for the retrenchment of our current era. It has become popular again to think of the cost of helping the poor as a major social problem.

What had happened to the notion that the poor, if given a chance, can and will solve their own problems—and that government can and should give them that chance? Part of the answer is that this notion of public responsibility competes in the public mind with a different, and very persistent, image. Upon researching the history of welfare debates, Katz writes,

> By the latter-nineteenth century poverty, crime, and disease blended to form a powerful, frightening, and enduring image. As is the case today, its dimensions were novelty, complexity, and danger. Among the urban poor, an undeserving subset, dependent on account of their own shiftless, irresponsible, immoral behavior, burdened honest taxpayers with the cost of their support, threatened their safety, and corrupted the working poor. Increasingly concentrated within slum districts, they lived in growing social isolation, cut off from the role models and oversight once provided by the more well-to-do, reproducing their own degradation. (1995, 68)

Katz points out that this model of poverty is still a dominant one in our politics, and that its effect is to focus discussion away from the structural causes of poverty (see chapter 4), toward the behavior of the poor themselves. Moreover, by erroneously portraying chronic inner city poverty as something new, the model lends strength to the arguments of conservatives who locate its causes in the liberal welfare laws enacted in the 1930s and 1960s.

For many decades, the role of the federal and state governments in relieving poverty has been under strong attack from fiscal conservatives. With the passing of postwar social optimism, this attack has gained ground. Since the 1970s, most states have not raised benefit rates, so that the effect of inflation has been to reduce the value of welfare payments, often to pre-1960 levels. At the same time, relief from state sources—General Assistance, as it is usually called—declined 32 percent between 1970 and 1985. The Reagan administration of the 1980s greatly reduced federal support for subsidized housing, a move that resulted in a major loss of income among the very poor (Katz 1989, 189). Federal subsidies for community health centers—a major source of health care to the poor—were also cut by 30 to 45 percent in 1982 alone, causing 239 centers to cut services or close (Dutton 1986). Some incentives for welfare recipients to work have been eliminated in an effort to reduce the AFDC roles. For example, the 1967 "thirty plus a third" rule, mentioned above, was dropped in 1981.

The Contract with America

The overriding conservative view of poverty, and of the role of the federal government in managing it, was well summarized in the Republican National Committee's widely circulated 1994 policy paper, *Contract with America* (Gingrich 1994). Let us summarize the welfare section of that paper (which also proposed cutting taxes while increasing spending for defense, police work, and prisons), and then turn to the incorporation of its thinking in the 1996 Budget Reconciliation Act—the current federal welfare policy.

> Isn't it time for the government to encourage work rather than reward dependency? The Great Society [referring to the welfare changes of the 1960s] has had the unintended consequences of snaring millions of Americans into the welfare trap. Government programs designed to give a helping hand to the neediest of Americans have instead bred illegitimacy, crime, illiteracy, and more poverty. Our Contract will achieve what some thirty years of massive welfare spending has not been able to accomplish: reduce illegitimacy, require work, and save taxpayers money. (Gingrich 1994, 65)

In these opening sentences of the welfare section, the *Contract* sets forth the essentials of its theory of poverty. Poverty is mainly a matter of individual choice, not social conditions, and welfare actually increases it (hence the title of the proposed legislation, The Personal Responsibility Act). Welfare itself creates incentives, not just to be idle, but to be irresponsible in other ways as well—having children out of wedlock, dropping out of school, and getting involved in illegal activities.

The choice of language, designed to symbolically associate government support of the poor with evil is most revealing. The malignant incentives of welfare are a "trap," so strong that many people find them irresistible. Unwed motherhood, largely the product of welfare, is one of the main causes of the tax burden. The children of unwed mothers are "illegitimate," by their existence an affront to society, and as such proof of the bad character of their parents. The real purpose of welfare is to give people a "helping hand," implying that anyone who is poor can be otherwise, and only those who are actively struggling deserve help. Federal spending on social services is described as "massive," an unacceptable burden. Such spending was actually 8.5 percent of U.S. gross national product in 1990—versus 23 percent for Great Britain and 34 percent for Sweden—but no such figures are given in the *Contract*. Nor are we told that in 1997, AFDC payments amounted to 1.17 percent of the federal budget (Nakao 1997, 3). All of this is wrapped in a tone of solicitousness toward the poor, intended to lull the reader's conscience to sleep while contemplating the effects of the proposed measures.

The main effects of the *Contract*'s section on welfare are

- To prohibit federal AFDC, housing, and food stamp payments to new categories of recipients: unwed mothers under eighteen; those who have not worked more than half time in the formal economy for five years. All categories of federal aid are denied to undocumented immigrants.
- To reduce the amount of AFDC payments to those who have children while on welfare.
- To delegate more authority (and cost) to states in spending federal money on welfare. For example, states may terminate welfare to unwed mothers under twenty-five, or those who have not worked for two years—even if one year was spent in a job training program. They may punish welfare recipients who have not finished high school. Control of health care and nutrition programs is delegated to the states as well.
- To end entitlements on all categories of federal welfare, and impose caps on the growth of welfare spending.
- To pass responsibility to the states for making the new guidelines work. States are required to design their own programs, for example, for moving welfare recipients into work. With the

end of entitlements, they are also required to work with fixed federal block grants, supplying whatever else is needed from their own budgets.

- To return savings on some programs to the states to be spent on services, not direct cash or in-kind payments to the poor.

These proposals, most of which became law by 1996, seem to be guided more by ideology than by attention to facts. The most glaring omission is any reference to the actual availability of jobs for which current and future welfare recipients might qualify. In the last chapter I discussed the actual availability of work. Also missing from the *Contract* are (a) any provision for services (child care, transportation, housing) that single mothers might need in order to stay in the formal economy as workers, and (b) any reference to a minimum income.

The failure of U.S. welfare "reform" to address the issue of job availability and job-support services is seen in clear relief if one contrasts the new policies with European responses to the problem of postindustrial unemployment. In Germany, the number of chronically unemployed people on welfare rose threefold, from .75 million to 2.4 million, between 1970 and 1987; but the response of the German government was very different from ours. Regulations were tightened, mainly to the disadvantage of foreign workers. But instead of simply cutting back the foreign labor supply, the Germans also offered inducements for citizens to leave the regular labor force—early retirement, or dignified alternative "work." Young men received subsidies for staying in school longer; women were paid to stay home and care for children and the elderly (Wilson 1993).

America's lack of attention to a minimum income is equally troubling. Most welfare recipients will have to accept jobs at, or near, minimum wage. The national average hourly wage for women entering a new job in 1992 was $5.07. For black teenagers it was $3.96. Working full-time year round, a mother of two children would have to earn $5.64 per hour to meet the 1992 poverty level (Smolensky et al. 1994, 19). A proposal that eliminates all welfare payments after five years, regardless of a family's income, then, must be seen not as a "helping hand," but as simple miserliness.

Moreover, actual scientific research on unwed parenthood, the central issue of the *Contract*, do not seem to incriminate welfare payments as the main cause, or even as an important factor. Since the mid-1970s, welfare payments have fallen steadily, whereas unwed pregnancies have not. The relationship between welfare payment rates in various states, and the rates of out of wedlock births in those states is also insignificant, as is the difference in the average size of welfare and nonwelfare families—1.9 children versus 1.8 (Smolensky et al. 1994, 25). I will return to this in a moment.

These are the most charitable things one can say about the *Contract*. If we look at it in the context of its likely long-term effects, a much harsher interpretation seems justified. Moving low-skilled workers into the labor force without systematically creating new jobs will almost certainly force wages down at the bottom end of the scale—according to the Economic Policy Institute as much as 12 percent. Early figures show disturbing trends: an estimated one thousand low-wage workers in Baltimore displaced by welfare "trainees" by early 1997 with another seventeen thousand welfare recipients likely to be pushed into the work force in subsequent months. In New York City at the same time there were thirty thousand welfare recipients doing public workfare jobs, thereby relieving the city of hiring regular workers (Cooper 1997, 12).

A secondary effect of this process is a kind of employment musical chairs, in which low-wage workers lose their jobs to trainees, go on welfare for a while, and then are recycled into the jobs of other laid-off workers. The resulting high turnover rates constantly cancels wage advances due to seniority, while also suppressing union membership, thereby further eroding wages and benefits. Like Sisyphus, the unskilled worker is repeatedly rewarded with consignment to the bottom of the climb. For now, we can only speculate about the effects of this on worker efficiency and productivity.

All of this of course improves corporate profits and accelerates the growing gap between rich and poor. It may help to account for the current (1997–1999) stock market boom, fueled by the unpredicted low inflation that accompanied vigorous economic growth. However, some parts of the *Contract* appear to be aimed less at upward economic redistribution than at simply mobilizing political sentiment. Loudly advertised cuts in payments to small, politically weak sectors of the poor—especially immigrants—actually have very little economic effect.

The Teenage Pregnancy Bag

Speaking in the Mississippi State Legislature in 1958, in favor a bill to sterilize unwed welfare mothers, State Representative David H. Glass said, "During the calendar year of 1957, there were born out of wedlock in Mississippi, more than seven thousand Negro children. . . . The Negro woman because of child welfare assistance [is] making it a business, in some cases, of giving birth to illegitimate children . . . The purpose of my bill is to stop, slow down, such traffic at its source" (quoted in Brown and Eisenberg 1995, 199–200). Mr. Glass's bill failed, but similar messages were heard in other legislative halls at the time, largely due to the increases in AFDC rolls following World War II that we have already noted. By 1974, an estimated one hundred thousand to one hundred and fifty thousand women of color were being sterilized annually under federally-funded programs (Brown and Eisenberg 1995, 199–200). The AFDC rolls have continued to grow, however, and Mr. Glass's message, in slightly more marketable language, has become a kind of mantra of the opponents of government spending on poverty. As the *Contract with America* makes clear, unwed pregnancy (by implication mostly teenage and black) is the centerpiece of the current attack on welfare. What are the facts?

Teenage pregnancy and birth rates are much higher in the United States than other industrial countries, and they are about twice as high among blacks as among whites. U.S. rates are going down among blacks, but they are going up overall, because more white teenagers are becoming pregnant, and blacks are only about 14 percent of our population. The Children's Defense Fund has estimated that only one in fifty-six poor children fit the popular stereotype of child poverty: poor black children in female-headed families in the inner city, on welfare, born to teenage mothers who don't work. (Aday 1993, 95). Unwed pregnancy rates are much higher among the poor than the nonpoor, but there are two flawed assumptions in the current attack on unwed motherhood as a cost-saving measure. The first wrong assumption is that cutting AFDC roles will save the American taxpayer a fortune. The second is that cutting AFDC will result in substantially lower rates of unwed pregnancy.

AFDC is not a large proportion of government spending, so even eliminating it will not result in the boon that the *Contract with America* approach suggests. Moreover, in their study of the California welfare system (10 percent of the nation's total), Smolensky and his colleagues show that decreases in AFDC are very unlikely to be recovered through the employment of single mothers. There are simply not enough jobs with adequate pay, and not enough services to keep them in what jobs there are. Their conclusions about the fiscal impact of requiring single mothers to work:

> AFDC isn't [eating up the budget], and nothing we are willing to do can make more than a marginal improvement in California's fiscal situation. . . . Clearly we should not pin our hopes for fiscal balance on further AFDC spending cuts. Besides, every dollar saved in AFDC spending is not necessarily a whole dollar saved, since some of the money spent on AFDC means less money spent on other "emergency" programs for the poor; to the extent that AFDC spending reduces the social costs of poverty, cuts in AFDC will be followed by increases in some other costs. (Smolensky et al. 1994, 27)

As for the second wrong assumption, as I mentioned above, research has failed to reveal any consistent influence of AFDC benefits on pregnancy rates. After an extensive review of the literature, Brown and Eisenberg conclude dryly, "In summary, the empirical literature does not lend support to the popular perception that AFDC and other income transfer programs exert an important influence on non-marital fertility" (1995, 198). The real reasons why single poor women have children is at least as complex as the reasons why men from ethnic ghettos find it hard to get and keep a job. Many writers speak of the low self-images of these women, and the rewards of prestige and affection that (they believe) will be theirs if they have children.

Others point to the fact that being *single* means different things in different cultures, and that many of the rewards for getting married have disappeared from poor communities where wider kin networks have always been at least as important as conjugal families. Where men cannot get reliable, legal work, where women are traditionally integrated into supportive kin networks, and where both sexes have come to expect a series of romantic relationships throughout their teenage and young adult years, marriage may tend to recede into the background as a goal for many. Carol Stack's ethnographic work among urban African Americans (see chapter 2) illustrates this. Whether or not the absence of a stable parental couple is harmful to children is an important issue, but it, too, is a complex one. Given the lack of evidence that welfare reduction leads to greater marital stability, it seems risky as an experiment in child psychology.

Still other studies show that high school culture in the United States today (no doubt urged on by media examples) puts an extreme emphasis on sexual attractiveness as a status measure, and that getting pregnant is the ultimate proof of success on this measure. Welfare cuts may, if anything, actually exacerbate some of these problems by further lowering the self-images and aspirations of low-income youth. Since it is unlikely that America will let unwed mothers and their children starve, the costs of feeding them will simply be shifted somewhere else.

Given the facts, the popularity of antiwelfare arguments based on the "welfare-momism" theory needs to be explained. One explanation is that the theory makes a certain rudimentary sense to those who are not really interested in the facts, but simply want lower taxes. In the mainstream media alternative proposals for cutting middle-class taxes get less coverage, for reasons I discussed in chapter 1. Military spending (somewhere between a quarter and a half of federal budget, depending on how you calculate it), tax breaks and subsidies for corporations and the wealthy, and social security and Medicare are sacrosanct.

But there is more to the popularity of the "welfare-momism" theory than the sheer lack of a competitor. It is rich in powerful symbols, and its proponents skillfully enlarge and embellish those symbols. From its Puritan foundations, the United States has inherited deep associations between sexual pleasure and evil. Those associations acquired an economic overlay during the industrial revolution. The new upward mobility of the middle-class family, together with declining infant mortality, suddenly meant that limiting fertility had major economic benefits. Children of small families could be educated, and education meant success. For the upwardly mobile young man or woman, an early and rigorous self-discipline in all matters, but especially in sex, became crucial. One need only read the advice meted out by educators and moralists of the Victorian Era to see the force of this complex. Both in order to conserve energy for study, and in order to cultivate a reputation that would ensure a "good" marriage, sex had to be suppressed. Sexual license assured poverty, and poverty in turn was a sign of unbridled sexuality. Church, where mere sexual thoughts were identified with Satan, was the training ground for middle-class morality. As sexual enjoyment was a sin requiring punishment, so poverty was God's punishment on earth of the promiscuous. No wonder that in such an environment, Freud discovered sexuality at the bottom of so much middle-class neuroticism.

Today we live in a sexually "enlightened" age, but these Victorian associations still haunt us on an unconscious level. Why do we still speak of eroticism as dirty? The word reveals the associations among sex, evil, and poverty. Why does the idea of school-based sex education, which has been shown to lower unwed pregnancy in many studies, still provoke moral outrage from large sectors of our communities? The acceptance of sexuality as a normal part of adolescence is still something terribly threatening to many. In American folklore and humor as well, the association between sexuality on the one hand, and skin color, social class, and education on the other hand, are close.

While few Americans, however liberal, would argue that single parenthood on a large scale is desirable, I think most would be willing to admit, on reflection, that in itself it does not prove moral degeneracy. But playing on our deep associations, the antiwelfare forces have carefully developed an iconography designed to suggest just that—a symbolism in which welfare dependency equals irresponsibility in general, and sexual promiscuity in particular. The word *illegitimacy* or its equivalent, *out-of-wedlock*, occurs six times in the first page-and-a-half of the *Contract with America's* section on welfare. In one place it is listed along with crime, illiteracy, and poverty as an effect of welfare. In another it is contrasted with *paternity and responsibility*, and it is the object of righteous reduction in one place, and attack in another.

An image is offered of the welfare recipient, then, that is as negative and as different as possible from the average person. The language seeks to evoke the deep fears and conflicts we have around sex, and by innuendo (without seeming vicious), to strengthen the ready association those fears have to our fears of the poor. To the extent that such iconography succeeds, clear thinking about welfare will become almost impossible, leaving the field to the we/they reflex, and counteracting whatever compassion we might be tempted to feel. The so-called religious right, for whom these fears are vibrantly conscious, constitutes one of the important constituencies of the antiwelfare bloc. Many in the religious right are poor or near-poor themselves—a fact that intensifies their need to disassociate from the icon of the welfare mom.[1]

Violence and Crime: Whose Problem?

Another claim of the welfare "reformers" is that America is experiencing an epidemic of violent crime, and that welfare is partly responsible for this. The *Contract with America* and other conservative analyses point out that crime rates and school dropout rates are higher in poor communities, and especially high among families on welfare. Their conclusion, in part, is that welfare itself produces family pathology, and hence poor educational performance, crime, violence, and drug use. Says conservative policy advisor Robert Rector (whose analyses form many of the key assumptions of the *Contract*): "[S]tudies confirm the negative effects of welfare on the development of children. For example, young women who are raised in families dependent on welfare are two to three times as likely to drop out and fail to graduate from high school than are [similar] women . . . not raised on welfare. . . . Boys raised in single-parent households are more than five times more likely to engage in criminal activity than are boys who are not raised in such conditions" (Rector 1995, 8). Similar conclusions are drawn by other conservative policy analysts (see Liebman 1995).

Studies do show that street crime (which actually has far less economic impact than white-collar crime) is in fact associated with economic inequality, and is higher in poor neighborhoods. It is difficult to find good statistics on actual rates of violence in the United States, since many of the official reports are for political reasons highly inflated (Kappeler, Blumberg, and Potter 1996, 35–38). Even so, we seem to have one of the highest rates of homicide in the world—7.9 per hundred thousand in 1984—more than seven times the rates of the British Isles, for example (Kappeler, Blumberg, and Potter 1996, 287). However, statistics do not support the notion that America is experiencing a crime wave. Contrary to the picture painted by the media, crime rates have dropped dramatically and continuously for the past two decades (Kappeler, Blumberg, and Potter 1996, 39). Historical studies of crime and violence tend to support the claim that they always accompany poverty and social disruption, and have not shown a general increase over time (Hawkins 1993).

The association of violence with drug use among the poor is highly distorted in the public imagination. Although there is indeed a relationship between drug use and violent crime, it is not clear what the relationship is—whether, for example, drug users become criminals or criminals become drug users. Ironically, the only drug that does seem to actually lead to criminal behavior is one that the power elite seems reluctant to discuss—alcohol (Kappeler, Blumberg, and Potter 1996, 174).

And yet one cannot read the ethnographies of inner city neighborhoods without being horrified by the level of violence that every careful observer finds there. What is new in the 1990s is the rising rate of homicide among inner city children and adolescents. A recent Detroit study of 246 Chicago youths between fourteen and twenty-three years of age found that 44 percent said they could access a gun within twenty-four hours; 42 percent had seen someone shot or knifed; 22 percent had seen someone killed; 18 percent carried a gun (Schubiner, Scott, and Tzelepis 1993). The number of actual killings tells only part of the story; the more serious part is the continuous fear both children and adults feel when they are surrounded by guns; where the slightest insult can result in the exchange of fire.

The etiology of this violence is hard to sort out. The continuous violence one finds on television and in films must play its part, as does the surprising availability of firearms and ammunition of all kinds. Again, in-depth discussion of these causes is rare in the mainstream media. The drug trade also plays a major role—by providing cash for weapons, by fostering criminal identities, by impairing the judgment of users, and by stimulating turf wars among dealers. In this book I am not so interested in tracing this complex etiology, as in providing a way of understanding the relationship of poverty and violence—a way that may be useful to the health worker.

Let us begin by examining the idea of violence.[2] First, because the idea provokes strong negative emotions, it is an important weapon in any ideological struggle, often out of all proportion to its actual prevalence or destructive effects. Ownership classes in most societies, including the United States, generally seek to focus on the physical violence associated with the poor because it distracts attention from the nonviolent forms of injustice typical of their own class. Kappeler et al. point out that white-collar crime is estimated to cost between 174 and 231 billion dollars annually in the United States—about seventeen times as much as all street crime combined (1996, 144).

Second, there is said to be such a thing as necessary violence, as in fighting an enemy or chastising a subordinate. The definition of what violence is necessary and what is not is again formed by those in power who have command over public opinion. But because even necessary violence is associated with evil (hence, necessary evil), if one is to use it to get and maintain power, one must do one's best either to disguise it as something else, or to legitimate it. Otherwise, the censure attending its use will negate one's efforts at persuasion (the other main source of power), and will ultimately elicit counterviolence from one's victims.

Accordingly, there is an intimate mutual relationship between political power, public discourse, and public image. I discussed this a bit in chapter 1, under "Maintaining the Status Quo." Other things being equal, the more power one has, the more influence one exerts over public discourse (the contents and forms of the media), and the better able one is to control one's public image.

By virtue of their wealth, corporations are able to present ideal-ized images of their products, services, and identities through ad-vertising; public officials fill the press with their rhetoric; priests and professors have access to their special audiences; and so on. The powerful are also able to disguise their violent behavior, exer-cising it through surrogates (the police and justice system) or pack-aging it in "soft" forms (the many forms of economic and political discrimination and manipulation) that seldom involve the use of physical force, but have the same effect. These soft forms of vio-lence, taken together, we generally refer to as *structural violence*.

The poor, of course, usually lack most of the means of man-aging their public image. At every level, from the personal to the international, the poor usually must rely either on pure persua-sion or on undisguised physical violence or the threat of same. In the game of image management, they are thus at a double disad-vantage: Not only do they lack the power to control public dis-course, but those who have that power are often their adversaries, using the media to delegitimize their efforts.

Add to this the commercial value of violence as a form of en-tertainment in a society that pays highly for stimulation, and one begins to recognize the context in which the violence of the poor is pushed forward. In short, the poor are often portrayed in pub-lic discourse as routinely disruptive and violent, or potentially so; while those who manage and profit from their exploitation, injury, insult, and slander—and their incarceration if they protest—are usually portrayed as far more peaceful.

The actual incidence of violence in the urban ghetto is far less, meanwhile, than we imagine. Bourgois points out that most inner city residents are rarely if ever victims of violence themselves— he himself lived in East Harlem for five years, and was only robbed once, in a store where everyone else was mugged at the same time. "Street culture's violence pervaded daily life in [this neighborhood] and shapes mainstream society's perception of the ghetto in a man-ner completely disproportionate to objective danger. Part of the reason is that violent incidents, even when they do not physically threaten bystanders, are highly visible and traumatic" (Bourgois 1995, 34).

I am not justifying violence of any kind, least of all that which the poor inflict on their own neighbors and kin, which I find appalling. What I am saying is that it loses some of its mystery and seems a bit more predictable once its context is understood. The residents of these poor neighborhoods are the daily victims of a structural violence whose effect is to shunt resources up the social scale, leaving them with inferior institutions, inferior housing, inferior pay, inferior public services, and inferior health. They know this. Meanwhile, their image as potentially dangerous is one of the few power cards they hold. As Piven and Cloward show (1971), the poor are most likely to advance as a class when they play that card collectively.

But with rare exceptions, most inner city violence involves individual-personal relations or youth gangs, and of course the great majority of poor do not participate at all. Even in Los Angeles, one of America's most gang-ridden cities, an estimated 90 to 95 percent of inner city youth do not belong to any gang (Stevens 1994). In chapter 2, I discussed how this kind of violence is romanticized in our culture, and how, in an environment of hopelessness, the warrior identity of some young working-class males lends itself to a kind of behavior that appears both self-destructive and cruel.

Many health care workers who elect to serve among the poor are overexposed to both the physical and emotional effects of drug use and violence, and this exposure adds greatly to the stress level of their work. The stress is made worse by the perception that this suffering is potentially avoidable, but beyond the knowledge and power of the health worker or victim to avoid or prevent. The sense of meaninglessness and powerlessness that arises from confronting something like this can be exhausting and depressing. I cannot offer a remedy of course, but in my own work I find the following ideas helpful:

- Although street crime is concentrated in inner city ghettos, there is actually far less violence among the poor than the media would have us believe.
- Physical violence in American society, while unacceptably high, is steadily declining.
- Although the effects of physical violence are dramatic and emotionally disturbing, the structural and legal violence of mainstream society is far more destructive on the whole.

- One is not completely helpless. Social and economic inequality is one of the major correlates of crime and violence; and people often unite to combat inequality once they understand its prevalence, its effects, and its mechanisms.

Comparison of the United States with a "Welfare State," Sweden

The American way of looking at the problems of poverty and the responsibility of government, then, is heavily conditioned by American culture, history, and politics. One way to understand this is to compare the U.S. system with a very different one from another equally affluent country. In choosing Sweden for such a comparison, my aim is not to prove how mean-spirited Americans are, but simply to show that what Americans take to be economically necessary or morally important is not given by any natural law.

It is difficult to make detailed comparisons between national welfare systems, because so many of the details of culture, history, and government differ from country to country, and these differences affect the way numbers translate into actual conditions. In traveling through northern Europe on a study tour of services for the elderly, for example, my wife and I found that living facilities for the aged in the Netherlands seemed emotionally warmer and more homelike than the more expensive and modern ones in Sweden. Statistics themselves can be misleading: Some European countries calculate the poverty level at half the median income, whereas the United States uses a measure of the cost of basic necessities. Given this caveat, here are some comparisons.

Philosophically, the Swedish government has been committed since 1969 to achieving gender and class equality, and full employment. To redistribute wealth, they rely on a relatively high, (about 40 percent) and highly progressive, set of taxes. In 1980, 23 percent of the average family's income was from welfare payments, and 5 percent of the population was poor, that is, received a total income of less than half the national median. The U.S. rate in 1997, calculated differently, was 13.3 percent (Census Bureau 1998).

Sweden gives priority in its welfare system to vulnerable populations such as single parents, the occupationally impaired, children, and the elderly. Pensions to the elderly are sufficient to assure that virtually no one over sixty-five is poor, in contrast to the United States, where the poverty rate among the elderly in general is 20 percent. If one is elderly, black, female, and living alone, the chances of being poor in this country are over 60 percent (Hess 1991, 10). In the strongly profamily and prochild Swedish welfare policy, there is an open attempt to level the socioeconomic playing field for children, whatever their birth status. In fact, in the 1980s, 35 percent of Swedish children were born outside of marriage, and 20 to 30 percent of families with children under eighteen were single parent. While the poverty rate of single parent families in the United States was 53 percent in 1987, the rate in Sweden was 5.5 percent (Ginsberg 1993; Rosenthal 1994). Ninety percent of Sweden's single parents are women, and 20 percent of single mothers receive welfare.

As part of the full employment policy, Sweden gives generous parental leave time to both married and single mothers, and provides generous child-care opportunities. Forty percent of single mothers are on welfare at any given time, but these mothers receive job training and housing subsidies as well as child care, and their average time on welfare is only four and a half months. Eighty-seven percent of all single mothers in Sweden work, and another 7 percent are in school (Rosenthal 1994).

The "Debate" on Health Care Policy

As I mentioned earlier, the welfare "debate" has been far from a mere academic exercise. Much of the conservative attack on welfare has been translated into law, largely through the Personal Responsibility and Work Opportunity Reconciliation Act of 1996. Since many details of administering the new federal policies are left to the states, it would be difficult to describe the effects of this law for the country as a whole. Let us, then, move from the national level to the local level to get an idea of the effects of the policy changes on the health care of the poor.

Since 1996, there are four main trends that are affecting health care of the poor: (1) the shift toward *capitation*, or prepaid contracts for Medicare and Medicaid payment; (2) changes in health care entitlement (who is eligible for what health services); (3) changes in entitlements for other benefits—cash, food, housing— that affect health status; and (4) strains on the health care delivery system resulting from these changes.

Capitation

Capitation is the growing tendency—not reflected in formal legislation—for health insurers, including Medicare and Medicaid, to seek to control their costs by signing *risk contracts* with health care providers (hospitals and clinics, physicians groups, HMOs, etc.), acting as *managed care providers*. A risk contract is simply an agreement, whereby the provider agrees to accept a flat yearly fee for each Medicare- or Medicaid-eligible patient, for whom it promises to provide a specified list of services. This practice (theoretically) saves the government money because the negotiated fee is generally less than the average cost of delivering health care to the patient population in question under cost reimbursement schemes. It helps the providers (again, in theory) because the patients must *enroll*, meaning they cannot go anywhere else for their primary health care unless they pay separately. Competition for the patients' insurance dollars is thereby eliminated. (In the grotesque parlance of managed care, enrolled patients are called *lives*, and the process of inducing them to enroll is called *capturing lives*.) Further, if the providers can reduce their cost per patient well below the capitated payment, they can make as much profit as they want.

By January 1998, over six million patients (16 percent of the total Medicare client population) were enrolled in Medicare managed care plans nationwide, and eighty thousand a month were joining such plans. By mid-1997, fifteen million Medicaid recipients (47 percent of the total) were also in managed care plans throughout the country (HCFA 1998, 2).

The impact this will have on the overall quality of health care to the poor is as yet unknown. Its advocates argue that the effect will be beneficial because providers will have to attract enrollees by offering them better services than their competitors. This is the point of the theory of health care financing called *managed com-*

petition. Detractors of the process point out several dangers. Capitation contracts provide an incentive for both insurers and providers to reduce costs wherever possible. This might have several effects. Under fee-for-service, providers were eager to have high-risk patients, since they expected to receive more insurance money for those who were sicker. Now providers try to discourage enrollment of high-risk patients, whose cost of care might run over the capitated amount. Once enrolled, high-risk patients may be discouraged from seeking the services they really need. Providers also seek to minimize costs and maximize profits by cutting staff, supplies, and services, resulting in lower quality care and enormous profits.

Both these problems pose a greater threat to the poor than to the affluent, for several reasons. First, affluent patients can afford to pay for extra services if those of their primary provider are inadequate. Second, wealthier patients tend to be the lower-risk patients—the patients most wanted by risk contractors. They have had better care all their lives; they are generally better educated and have better health habits; they live and work in healthier and safer environments; and they have the knowledge, transportation, and help needed to access the care system earlier and more often. They also tend to have more access to informal supports, such as family (Ware et al. 1996).

At this writing, managed care HMOs have already begun to cut programs for the poor and the elderly from their services. Large firms like Aetna, U.S. Healthcare, Pacificare, Oxford Health Plans, Kaiser Permanente, and Blue Cross and Blue Shield have shut down medicaid serivces in at least twelve states, including New York, New Jersey, Florida, Massachusetts, and Connecticut. Meanwhile, HMOs that serve elderly Medicare patients are also beginning to close these down. Twenty counties in Ohio were served by Anthem Blue Cross Blue Shield until May 1998, when the program was dropped, leaving hundreds of elderly patients without the services they had come to rely on. The same month the large HMO Health Net also closed its Medicare program in ten California counties (Kilborn 1998).

An even greater threat to the poor from capitation is the reduction of Medicaid payments, as state agencies play one provider off against another. Under current Medicaid capitation schedules, providers are unable to sustain many preventive and screening services (see "Facilities Serving the Poor" below).

Another danger of capitation is that high-quality providers and those that specialize in services to the poor and high-risk may be either forced out of business, or required to join larger conglomerates with lower standards, as insurers negotiate lower payments to larger HMOs. The system favors large, corporate systems over private practitioners and small neighborhood clinics because the larger systems can (a) influence state policy by heavy lobbying; (b) negotiate lower fees due to savings of scale; (c) mobilize capital for advertising and cosmetic changes to plant. Most community-owned and operated clinics for the poor in California, for example, have had to join provider networks that include other providers who have never specialized in service to the poor, and probably have inferior skills in meeting their needs. The state of California has already shifted to risk contracting of Medicaid in thirteen counties, and the contracted fees and coverages are well below fee-for-service levels.

Still another criticism of capitation is that it produces high administrative costs. Most providers lack the skills and facilities needed to negotiate capitation contracts, monitor and control costs, locate and recruit patients, and a host of other complex nonmedical tasks that come with managed care. These providers typically have to contract with a management firm for such services, and the manager's fees are taken out of the patients' insurance payments, thereby lowering the percentage of the payment that goes to actual care.

These criticisms are not simply the carping of a medical Luddite. Almost daily one hears horror stories about what happens to people under managed care. Here are some recent ones gathered from the author's own classes, reading, and casual encounters:

- Nurse Rhonda Burton works for a community clinic in Richmond. A child who broke his foot could not get the bone set because the only orthopedic specialist willing to see the patients of this clinic, who are all low-income, lives in Dublin—some

45 miles away. The pediatrician had to call his orthopedist friends one by one and beg them to see the child free of charge.

- The priest at St. Luke's Church in Berkeley is elderly and needs a kidney transplant. His sister has offered to donate her kidney, and the physicians are ready to do the procedure, but his insurance company has delayed week after week to authorize the operation. He thinks they are waiting for him to die.

- Nurse Joyce Beck's husband gets care at an HMO in San Jose. He recently had to have an operation, with full anesthesia. Following the procedure he was wheeled on a gurney into the "recovery area," which was actually a hallway with ample foot traffic. He was given a beeper and told to call if he needed anything. Joyce couldn't stay with him, because she had to go to her job.

- Nurse Carolyn Lee, working in a large HMO, saw a family bring in a member suffering from tachycardia. After he had waited for two hours, a physician listened to his heart and prescribed digoxin. No other diagnostic or monitoring procedures were requested.

- Another nurse in one of my classes had spoken with a physician from a "large managed care organization," who told her patients with coronary artery disease are often denied surgery and managed with medication, when in fact their disease is very advanced. When she pointed out that the organization would lose money when these patients ended up in the ICU, he said, "We count on these patients with severe CA disease to die before reaching the hospital."

- The *Wall Street Journal* of May 30, 1997 describes the following string of incidents: In August 1994 . . . an elderly homeless man who was disoriented entered the Sunrise [a Las Vegas hospital of HMO chain Columbia/HCA] emergency room; it discharged him without performing a CAT scan. Hours later, he ended up at a Catholic hospital, which ran a scan and found a brain hemorrhage that required surgery. Sunrise refused to take him back.

  The case resulted in an inquiry by the federal Health Care Financing Administration, which received a "Patient Dumping" complaint. A HFCA report shows that the agency looked at Sunrise records and found that on the same day, another Sunrise patient with similar symptoms—but with insurance coverage—received a battery of tests and was admitted. Sunrise lost its Medicare certification but won a reprieve after promising to make reforms, such as an education program for emergency room workers.

Still, several months later another homeless man was denied treatment at the Sunrise emergency room, according to [the hospital's former vice president]. He said that a doctor gave the man a glass of juice and noted on his chart that he was "filthy" and suffering from "acute homelessness." He was ushered out. About an hour later, the man died of pneumonia on the hospital lawn.

Health Care Entitlements

The federal government's Personal Responsibility and Work Opportunity Reconciliation Act of 1996 makes four kinds of changes in eligibility for welfare. It (1) replaces federal guarantees with fixed sums payable to states; (2) eliminates certain categories of recipients; (3) adds eligibility restrictions on recipients; and (4) caps lifetime benefits.

Again, the actual effects of these changes on the health care of the poor are not yet clear, but have begun to play out after July 1, 1997, when the act took effect. In place of federal guarantees based on national standards of eligibility and payment, the government now sets broad guidelines that must be met by states in order to receive federal welfare funds. States may set stricter criteria, as in the California plan. Since Medicaid is decoupled from welfare under the federal law, welfare recipients will lose their Medicaid rights until their state redetermines their eligibility for SSI and AFDC (now called TANF) separately. At the very least, this meant a gap of several months in coverage for thousands in mid-1997, during which health services to the poor experienced some chaos. At the worst, it meant elimination of many categories of recipients formerly eligible. Those disqualified are SSI recipients with drug and alcohol problems; pregnant undocumented alien women; all legal aliens; those with federal drug convictions; children over fourteen with mild disabilities; and most SSI and TANF recipients who fail to get work within a specified time.

Undocumented aliens were already excluded from federal welfare programs, but states and localities had the option of providing services to them. California, which has historically provided prenatal and maternity care to illegal immigrants, adopted anti-alien legislation that eliminates that benefit, and requires health workers to report undocumented patients. In December of 1997, a court injunction against that law was upheld.

Some of those formerly covered under Medicaid (for example, the elderly and disabled) continue to receive Medicare as well. Others have lost their only health insurance, limiting their access to charity care and emergency rooms. In mid-1999, this number was estimated at 675,000, most of them children (Wellstone 1999).

Income Entitlements

Probably the largest impact of welfare reform on health will result from the loss of income and in-kind support for food and housing. (Incidentally, loss of health insurance will also constitute loss of income, for those who must pay out of pocket for health services.) Many studies show that poverty per se is closely correlated with ill health.

The new law eliminates SSI coverage for most legal aliens who lack substantial work histories, and gives states the option of cutting their other benefits as well. This is aimed mainly at relatives of Johnson Act immigrants, many of whom are elderly and now receive Medicaid as well as Medicare. California might keep benefits for those already here, but eliminate them for new legal immigrants.

Changes in eligibility for AFDC, SSI, food stamps, and related services such as subsidized housing, mean that many individuals and families will lose some or all of their benefits if they cannot meet work or other requirements within the specified time limits. Most of these may lose their Medicaid eligibility after a grace period yet to be determined (see above). Most of those who continue to receive welfare benefits will receive less. The federal law reduces grants to states by 15 percent below 1995 levels. The food stamp program has been cut $28 billion, reducing payments per meal from $0.80 to an estimated $0.66.

The burden of providing jobs, housing, and other essential services to this new destitute population falls on county and local governments. Most California county and city budgets for health care to the indigent are already strained to the breaking point, and the additional indigent caseload is expected to bring about a widespread decay of this system. It is widely feared that states will worsen the situation over the long term, by engaging in competitive tax- and benefit-cutting to attract industry and jobs—the so-called race to the bottom.

One issue seldom discussed with respect to entitlements, is the loss of activity in the economy that will result from the reduced income of the poor. According to one estimate, the $28 billion cut in food stamps will result in the loss of seven hundred thousand jobs in the food industry. Similar losses can be expected in other basic industries that provide goods and services to the poor—everything from barbering to Wal-Mart stores. Another neglected issue is that of income depression. Millions of unemployed scrambling for the lowest-paying jobs is certain to have a depressive effect on wages at the lower levels. As wages at the lower margin fall (in the absence of a decent minimum wage) many families that are now one step away from disaster will cross the line, creating a new army of people in need of public support. The best jobs for those now on welfare are likely to go to recipients who already have education and skills, and would have soon been employed in any case. No federal agency currently tracks former welfare recipients to see how they are faring. Incidentally, too, dire necessity is likely to increase crime, an effect that will make further demands on overstressed community budgets.

Health Facilities Serving the Poor

The impact of these entitlement and funding changes on health facilities serving the poor is likely to be serious. Loss of access to preventive and primary care is likely to result in greatly increased use of high-cost emergency services. Many facilities that now serve primarily low-income populations, such as community clinics and county hospitals, are losing large shares of income from public re-imbursements. Both these developments will mean poorer health *and* higher costs of care to the poor and uninsured near-poor. Community clinics are able to serve the uninsured near-poor at little or no cost because they (a) raise funds from donations, endowments, grants, and local public health funds as well as fees; (b) operate with low overhead, in areas where frills are unnecessary; and (c) spread overhead costs over large insured patient populations. As clinics lose clients and accept lower reimbursements for care, they will either have to close—shifting the burden of care to other providers—or raise client copayments, to cover more of their costs.

The East Boston Health Center is one example. The center serves an overwhelmingly low-income population with about three hundred thousand visits in 1997. The area's average annual income is less than fifteen thousand dollars, and in 1998, 23 percent of the clinic's patients were uninsured. The State of Massachusetts has a fund meant to reimburse hospitals for the costs of serving the uninsured, but in 1998 that fund only covered about 60 percent of hospitals' outlay. That year the East Boston Health Center, a community health center founded in 1970, found itself with ten million dollars in disallowed expenses for uninsured care, and as of this writing (March 1999) is faced with closing (Daniel 1999).

In another example, 60 percent of the visits at Berkeley Primary Care Access Clinic, a community clinic serving a low-income clientele, are uninsured. The clinic charges a minimum fee (to anyone who can pay) of fifteen dollars per visit. In order to stay open under the coming regime, where they stand to lose 20 to 30 percent of their patients who are Medicaid insured (AFDC, SSI, GA, and the like), they have had to raise their fees to the uninsured. In order to retain services for the uninsured, in March 1999 the clinic had to open a night facility staffed by volunteer providers.

Meanwhile, as we have mentioned, county-supported facilities for the indigent will also suffer a loss of income from the same sources, and in addition will have to spread revenues over a much wider range of needs, as the poor lose income and in-kind benefits, and as new needs for job training, child care, and subsidized work emerge from the new requirements.

The "worst case" scenario, then, is one of a cascade of effects, in which not only the current welfare population falls through the shredded safety net and becomes destitute, but a new class of needy is created by the resulting strain on both the public and private sectors; with resulting increases in remedial costs—for emergency medicine and psychiatric care, crime control and prisons, emergency food and housing, and remedial education. The worst case will probably not come to pass, simply because communities will respond with compassion and creative vision as they always have. But avoiding the worst case will be a monumental job, for all of us.

Needed: A New Kind of Debate

Exposing the staleness and sterility, the willful ignorance, and the shabby salesmanship of the conservative-led "debate" on welfare and health care policy is only a first step. Liberal writers have been doing that since the beginning of the current attacks. In fact, against these attacks, the liberal intellectuals generally argue that their policies have had many good effects, and that with some adjustments they can be made to work better. They point to the success of Head Start in improving the performance of low-income children in school, and plead for greater investment in education at all levels (Katz 1989, 21; Smolensky et al. 1995, 49). They show that poverty rates decreased dramatically among the highest risk groups—children, the elderly, and minorities—due to income transfer programs and improved educational opportunities during the liberal era of the 1960s and 1970s (for example, Katz 1989, 242). They argue that job training programs like JOBS, initiated in 1988, have shown promise, but languish for lack of funding.

These liberal arguments do not seem to be having much effect on welfare policy in the 1990s, either at the national or the state levels. Part of the problem is that they are not well represented at the highest levels of power, either official or unofficial. Liberal politicians, well aware that real welfare reform would cost real money, have been reluctant to identify themselves with it in an era of tax revolt. The popular media have little incentive to publicize it, given the politics of the owners and advertisers of television and the press.

Accordingly, advocates of a strong state role in welfare naturally tend to be absorbed by the problem of restoring, protecting, and extending what they see as the gains of earlier policies. Especially those involved in the day-to-day lives of the poor at the personal and community level, see the real suffering brought on by the new harsher atmosphere, and are swept up in the effort to hold the line against its worst effects. In doing so, they often neglect the task that alone may eventually produce large and lasting results: To challenge forcefully the basic concepts and language of the public discussion, in order to refocus it on what we know about the real causes of poverty.

As we have seen in this book, the main causes of poverty are the shunting of wealth upward in the class hierarchy, and the increasing geographic and social isolation of the poor in deteriorating environments. I believe that the vast majority of Americans would like to see both these processes reversed, up to a point; the question is how to empower people to begin the work of reversing them.

The obstacles to that work are enormous, but not insurmountable. Behind these causes of poverty lies a political process that links power closely with wealth and severely hinders ordinary people's efforts to organize around their own interests. This political process is sustained (a) by the control of the mainstream media by the financial elite, which assures that only ideas acceptable to the wealthy get a serious hearing, (b) by the closed loop of political success, in which few get elected without access to wealth; and (c) because few who challenge the system have access to wealth.

One of the results of this arrangement is the device of the two-party system. Having two parties assures that all political battles will be over the middle ground of politics, the uncommitted voters who might be persuaded that there is a real basis for a choice. In multiparty parliamentary systems, candidates tend to build constituencies around strong positions on controversial issues, and fight for the right to represent those positions in a pluralistic government.

American Democrats and Republicans, by contrast, seek to avoid controversial ideas, for fear of taking a position that turns out to be less popular than the other party's. Having promised only measures known to have a large constituency, the winners then feel free to change their positions according to the latest polls. Although elected office holders might have long-term agendas, their short-term activities are calculated mainly to keep them out of trouble. In the absence of a party with a clear and consistent social vision, voters elect personalities instead of platforms, and those elected may vote as they choose without fear of party discipline.

This regime is extremely stable for two reasons: First, as I said, the existing parties retain control of the resources needed to attract public attention. Given their aversion to controversy, they will generally keep truly innovative ideas out of the media. Second, the very lack of a clear platform leaves both parties free to co-opt the language of any new idea that actually manages to surface in the public consciousness. The substance of this idea is then subjected to the art of political compromise, until its more innovative aspects have been softened. A familiar example is the issue of patient's rights under managed care. To confront the systemic evil—the fact that cutting quality is rewarded in a prepaid, profit-driven system—would risk the wrath of big corporate medicine. Legislators prefer to appease public outrage by tinkering with fraud and abuse disclosure bills.

For the foreseeable future at least, this is the political context within which health workers interested in the conditions of the poor must operate. The strategies that they choose by which to improve their effectiveness must be crafted for this environment. The ground covered by the welfare and health care "debate" is not going to shift quickly. Without strenuous and constant pressure from articulate advocates of the poor, it is unlikely to shift at all.

Given the social role and public image of the health care professions, a variety of strategies might be effective, and I have neither the experience nor the imagination to list them. Here are some of the resources that concerned health workers might draw on, and some suggestions about their strategic value.

- *Humanitarianism*: The essentially humanitarian nature of health care work gives professionals some credibility when they speak on behalf of disadvantaged groups. Although there is currently considerable cynicism in America about this humanitarian image, I believe there is also a good deal of faith in it. Portrayals of health workers in the media are mostly positive in this regard.

- *Science*: As well trained professionals, health workers (a) generally are seen as people who speak from knowledge, at least when it comes to health (an image that is supported by the media; and (b) actually do have a large repertoire of both factual data and analytic skills they can use in public debate.

- *Social Class*: Although many health professionals, particularly nurses, come from working-class backgrounds, the public image of the health professional is middle class. This is the "good news" side of the fact that most Americans discriminate morally in favor of that class.

- *Peer Solidarity*: Although there are dramatic political differences among health professionals, as in any profession, there is also a potential for solidarity in the professional courtesy extended by members of a particular discipline (medicine, nursing, midwifery, physical therapy, mental health, etc.) to one another. Like-minded health workers have a social basis for forming cooperative groups among themselves. Good liberal examples of this are Physicians for Social Responsibility and Physicians for Human Rights.

- *Access to Information*: Health professionals are accustomed to dealing with a high volume of complex information in many forms. Most have access to and familiarity with electronic and published reports and data sets. Many are also skilled in data collection and analysis methods, such as interviewing, observation, and statistical applications.

- *Communication Skills*: Good clinical practice requires excellent communication skills—although I hasten to add that more than a few health workers could use some improvement in this area. Political advocacy, like health care, benefits from the ability to make complex material clear and persuasive to the average person.

This "cultural capital" can be used to force the inclusion of useful information about poverty and health into the public debate.

Readers will already know about a number of techniques, such as letter writing, joining advocacy groups, serving on boards and commissions, and attending open public forums. One can emphasize one's professional status in all of these. Most activities can be greatly enhanced by

- keeping an up-to-date *file of facts* that can be used to support arguments. Sources of data on poverty and health are included in Appendix A of this book.
- *budgeting time* to devote to advocacy. Unprotected time usually gets spent on matters of immediate concern—advocacy is usually slow and long-term.
- doing what health workers usually call *outreach*—looking for inactive people who are interested in the problem and may be willing to help with the task. This can mean anything from casually starting conversations with co-workers, to searching the internet, to reading the letters section of your local newspaper and contacting the writers, to actually canvassing your workplace or community.
- establishing robust *communication links* with like-minded people, especially activists, both within and outside one's profession. Such links can provide mutual motivation and support, broaden knowledge, and multiply efforts through better coordination.

The demands of work and domestic life on the socially conscious health worker are typically great. Most of us feel we are not participating in the debate as much as we should. Perhaps our best contribution is to give ourselves credit for, and take pride in, whatever we are able to do. Advocacy is not only a legitimate part of health care practice, but it is also an indispensable part of citizenship in a democratic society.

Exercises and Study Questions

1. Find a recent mainstream news article on poverty and health care reform. What facts and issues form the focus of the story, and what is left out?

2. Talk to a *middle-class* unwed parent—or rent the film *Antonia's Line*. How does social class affect the experience of unwed parenthood and single-parent childhood?

3. Imagine you are jobless. You never went to college, you have no skilled job experience, and you have exhausted your unemployment and welfare benefits. Neither you nor your relatives nor friends have savings or assets (car, computer, house, business, welfare, pension, investments, and so forth). Figure out how to eat and pay rent between now and the end of next month, when your landlord will evict you for nonpayment.

4. You are on the board of a foundation that gives one million dollars per year to support projects aimed at improving "equity in health access." What kind of projects will you look for?

5. If asked, what would you recommend to a congressional group drafting legislation on basic health care reform?

The Poor under the Stethoscope
Health and Health Care

When I set out to write this chapter, my idea was to present a comprehensive overview of the health problems that poor people have, in order to alert students to the kind of medicine/ nursing/public health they need to learn in order to work effectively in poor communities. Once I got into the statistics on the health of the poor, I realized that the numbers on rates of illness and disability may not be helpful at all. It is a fact that the health of poor people as a group is worse than that of the nonpoor—usually measured by rates of death, diagnosed illness, and disability. All the major sources of aggregate health data tell us the poor have—and have had for a long time—more cancer, arthritis, heart disease, tooth and gum disease, diabetes, respiratory disease, vision and hearing problems, psychiatric problems, more days of missed work due to sickness and disability, higher rates of HIV infection, and earlier deaths than the nonpoor. As one pair of epidemiologists put it, "In summary, persons in lower-class groups have higher morbidity and mortality rates of almost every disease or illness, and these differentials have not diminished over time" (Syme and Berkman 1976, 3). The poor are sicker when first seen by a doctor, they smoke more, and their nutrition and hygiene is poorer. Most of these observations also distinguish nonwhites from whites, but these distinctions generally disappear when races are compared at the same income level.

Without explanation, this in itself tells the health worker little about how to approach a poor community. The problem is that no one seems to know much about the causes of class-related illness rates. In the pages that follow, I consider the most important factors that might help to understand the dynamics of illness and disability among the poor, from a health care point of view. These are

- *The chicken/egg question*: To what extent is illness caused by poverty, and to what extent is poverty caused by illness?

- *The behavioral/environmental question*: Does the ill health of the poor stem more from disease, resulting in turn from psychosocial vulnerability, stemming from their emotional situation (stress, depression, lack of social support, feelings of helplessness, and so on), from their less effective knowledge, beliefs, and practices (medical knowledge, hygiene, risk behaviors, communication skills, and the rest), or from their physical situation (sanitation, shelter, work and environmental hazards, nutrition, access to care, health practices, and so on)?

- *The responsibility question*: To what extent, and in what sense, is the health of the poor the responsibility of society, of the family, or of the individual?

- *The intervention strategy question*: How, if at all, can resources be allocated with maximum effect to improve the health of the poor?

Causal Relationships in the Ill Health of the Poor

It may seem fairly obvious that the relationship between poverty and ill health is not a simple case of which causes which, but of how much of the one can be accounted for by the other. Being poor certainly adds to the stress, both physical and psychological, of most low-income people, and reduces their access to many sources of wellness such as knowledge, a wholesome environment, and the ability to buy top quality services. At the same time, sickness both limits one's ability to get a living—through either the formal or the informal economy—and burdens one with costs that well people do not have. There seem to be two main points of view on the chicken or egg question in the literature: (a) most poverty can be explained by illness; (b) poverty is an intervening variable that helps to explain illness rates: that is, whatever the cause of illness, poverty is a factor that increases its frequency and severity, and makes recovery more difficult. The distinction among these points of view is more than merely academic, because each suggests a different way of attending to the health problems of the poor.

A good example of position (a) is Luft's (1978) study of health and income. Luft notes that social spending on the health of the poor has been aimed mainly at improving their access to the same kind of high-tech medicine enjoyed by the nonpoor, and that this has not been effective. Noting that poor people are generally sicker when they first see a doctor than the nonpoor are, and that they have dramatically higher rates of disability, he concludes that having a relatively incurable condition often results in the severe restriction of the individual's ability to find well-paid work. This fact, when added to problems of low education, racial and sex discrimination, and lack of other resources, then condemns many people to poverty. "At least 30 percent of the disabled who are currently poor," says Luft, "are poor *because* of their health problems; among white men this figure is close to 75 percent. Disability is responsible for 9 to 18 percent of *all* poverty among the non-aged. Similarly, at least 23 to 31 percent of all non-aged poor white men are poor because of their disability" (8). He notes moreover that welfare payments "total only about 40 percent of the lost earnings [due to disability] and remove from poverty only 40 percent of the disabled who were impoverished by health problems" (8). Finally, Luft concludes that "relatively few people who would otherwise be healthy are sick *simply because they are poor*" (15; his emphasis).

The implications of Luft's viewpoint are fairly clear. If disability could be prevented, through better health education, occupational safety, improved sanitation and housing, and other public health measures such as screening and immunization, a sizable proportion of the population would cease to be poor. More attention to physical and occupational rehabilitation would decrease the poverty census even more.

In my view, there is a good deal of useful information in Luft's study, and his suggestions for reform are well worth while. Still, I am less optimistic that his program would have a major effect either on the incidence of poverty, or on the health of the poor. The largest problem with his analysis is that it assumes the availability of well-paid jobs for the able bodied—a flawed assumption, which I have dealt with in chapters 4 and 5. Although there is no denying an association between poverty and disability, that association would seem to be an extremely complex one, in which factors such as the availability of any kind of work plays a major part. Being out of work though healthy, for example, leads to a willingness to accept more dangerous working and living conditions, which in turn raises rates of disability. It also leads to more work in the informal economy (extra-legal manufacturing and services, bootleg labor, child labor, prostitution, barter economy, and so on) where products and work conditions are largely unregulated.

Another difficulty is that the data on poverty and health do seem to indicate major nondisabling problems, and major problems in children and youth, that can scarcely be attributed to their diminished earning ability. Luft's own statistics, for example, show that in children between six and seventeen years of age, poverty is associated with worse hearing and more hearing abnormalities, more decayed and missing teeth, less filled teeth, more periodontal disease and worse oral hygiene, less height, weight, and skeletal maturity, and higher blood pressure. One is tempted to say that Luft has reached his conclusions by extrapolating from a definition of *unwellness* to mean disabled adulthood.

Writers who take the position that poverty is an intervening variable that contributes to illness rates, differ with respect to the *behavioral/environmental question*; that is with respect to the way they think poverty contributes to ill health. Some, such as Adler et al. (1993), acknowledge environmental factors, but emphasize the emotional, cognitive, and behavioral correlates of being poor—

stress, lack of knowledge, and poor hygiene. Others, such as Aday (1993), Yee and Capitman (1996), and Doyal (1979), take the more environmental viewpoint—that being poor imposes physical and social conditions on whole populations that in and of themselves guarantee higher rates of illness.

Not surprisingly, the choice of emphasis generally follows the discipline of the observer: Adler is a psychologist, Doyal a political economist, and Aday, Yee, and Capitman are health policy analysts. In justifying the behavioral approach, Adler et al. begin by noting two facts. (a) The relationship of health to income is not dichotomous (poor = bad health; nonpoor = good health), but follows a continuum: mortality and morbidity are inversely related to income at all levels, including the highest. (b) This relationship holds not only in countries like the United States, where access to healthy surroundings and medical care is clearly related to employment and income, but to a smaller degree also in countries like Sweden and Great Britain, where such access is, theoretically at least, tolerably equal across classes. The relationship, then, must be largely due to nonenvironmental factors. The psychologists suggest an array of causes that includes emotional burden (*life stress* and *lack of resilience*) and thinking and behavioral habits, such as the way events and conditions are perceived (*appraisal*) and dealt with (*coping skills*). They also mention *situational obstacles* to care, such as time, distance, and access to technology.

This view is roughly the epidemiological equivalent of the "culture of poverty" position that has been popular in policy circles since the 1960s. As I mentioned in chapter 3, there is undoubtedly some merit in the view that norms of thinking and behaving vary according to economic class, and it would be very surprising if these differences had nothing to do with health. Direct observation of health care settings (see Duff and Hollingshead 1968; Kozol 1994) confirms that the poorer one is, the less likely one is to (a) have faith in a system run by an educated elite; (b) have the communication skills, self-confidence, and knowledge to access the health care system easily; and (c) be able to negotiate good care and make maximum use of information once one has accessed the system.

Counterpoint: Access to Care

On the other hand, to limit attention to the psychological dimensions of poverty would be to overlook much of the problem. The same studies that show the handicaps of the poor in dealing with the health care system also show the dramatic bias of the American health care industry, at all levels, in favor of the well-to-do. There are really two issues involved in assessing this bias: the issue of access to care, and the issue of quality of care. The interactions of poverty with these factors are difficult to measure, but one can get some idea of the effects of poverty on access by looking at the problems of the uninsured and those on Medicaid. First, the uninsured:

- About 40 million Americans, most of them working poor, have no health insurance. Rates of noninsurance are higher for blacks than whites, and highest of all for Hispanics (extrapolating from Bodenheimer and Grumbach 1997, 19).
- The rate of noninsurance among those with incomes below 125 percent poverty in 1989 was 27 percent. Among those with incomes over $25,000, the rate was about 7 percent (Bodenheimer and Grumbach 1997, 23).
- Despite the common perception that urgent care, at least, is available to anyone who wants it in the United States, people with health insurance receive 90 percent more hospital services, and see a doctor 70 percent more often than those without insurance (Bodenheimer and Grumbach 1997, 25).
- Health outcomes are worse for the uninsured than the insured. They have more avoidable hospitalizations, are sicker when seen by a doctor, have lower birth weight babies, and have twice the mortality rate of the insured (Bodenheimer and Grumbach 1997, 26–27).

Poor people on Medicaid fare somewhat better than the uninsured in getting access to health services, but not as well as those with private insurance. Moreover, only about half of U.S. families with incomes below federal poverty guidelines are eligible for Medicaid, and even those who are eligible face problems.

- In 1991, 61 percent of U.S. physicians either did not accept Medicaid payments for services, or restricted the number of Medicaid patients in their practice. In a 1992 survey, 18 percent of nonelderly Medicaid patients reported that they had been refused services (Bodenheimer and Grumbach 1995, 27).
- Some studies show more advanced illness at diagnosis or hospital admission among Medicaid than privately insured patients (Bodenheimer and Grumbach 1997, 28).

Ethnographic details help to make these issues concrete. Kozol details how middle-class hospitals in New York sometimes refuse to treat low-income patients.

> "Three years ago," says one of the grandmothers who prepare the meals for the soup kitchen at St. Ann's, "I was having bad pains in my breast and my right arm. I went to Mount Sinai because I had a bad experience at Lincoln.
>
> "'You live in the South Bronx. Your catchment area is Lincoln Hospital,' they said. 'Why don't you go back there in your own zone?' I said, 'I have Medicaid.' They said, 'We can't help you.'" (1995,178)

Counterpoint: Quality of Care

The quality of health care is, as I said, difficult to measure, but the idea that the health care industry fulfills its goal of giving equal services without reference to income is, to say the least, questionable. For over a century, many of our poor have received their medical care from teaching hospitals, where they have often been treated more or less as lab specimens. In their landmark study of such a hospital in the 1960s, Duff and Hollingshead contrasted the conditions on the open wards—where low-income patients were seen—with those in the private and semiprivate rooms reserved for the more affluent:

> The ward accommodations were outstanding in several ways in the matter of the fears of the patients: Ward patients were the poorest, sickest, and most crowded in the hospital. They were cared for by a rushed group of physicians and nurses,

who, under the circumstances, showed little concern for them beyond care for the physical condition. These patients were generally deprived socially. Their hospital care reflected and extended that deprivation. More than patients in other accommodations, they harbored terrifying memories and suspicions which were then added to their long list of life's adversities. While fears of illness and treatment and life misfortunes where found in all groups, the situation for the ward patients was the most trying. Accustomed as they were to adversity, ward patients found their accommodations oppressive. (1968, 286)

The extreme suspicion toward the physicians shown by the ward patients was not unfounded. Doctors rarely told the patients what was happening to them, avoided emotionally charged issues, and were not interested in their social conditions. Thirty years later, these findings are borne out by other studies: "Research consistently shows that less information from physicians about conditions, positive lifestyle changes that could improve or modify conditions, and less communication overall is provided to low-income patients and those of color than to those with higher incomes" (Yee and Capitman 1996, 260). Yee and Capitman also note that women get fewer procedures for coronary heart disease than men do, and that there are fewer follow-ups on cancer diagnosis for nonwhite than for white patients.

Nor are the institutions equivalent in poor and nonpoor communities: "[M]any inner city hospitals are financially distressed. Several institutions closed down during the past decade, and many survivors now face multiple adverse trends. These include the continued scarcity of physician practices in inner cities and the denial of services to inner city patients by many primary physicians. These developments tend to increase the severity of illness of care seekers in inner city institutions" (Gautam et al. 1995, 388). Kozol puts it this way:

David's mother [an African American who has cancer and lives on welfare in the South Bronx] goes to the hospital again in February. This time, she's held for four nights in a downstairs corridor before a bed is free.

"I took her there on Monday," David tells me on the

phone. "It was one of those bad nights. We got there at seven, but it was so crowded there was no place to lie down. She sat up for five hours. Then at midnight I went to a nurse and said she needed to lie down.

"The nurse got mad and snapped at me. She said, 'I can't grant your request.' My mother had to sit there until 3 A.M. At three they put her on a stretcher and a doctor looked at her. He said she needed x-rays but he said there was no one free to do them. She didn't get the x-ray for two days.

"She spent another three nights down there on the stretcher in the hallway. When they finally found a room for her she suddenly began to shiver and her hands were cold. They didn't have no blankets." (1995, 98)

These conditions are not new. Of the hospital outpatient departments and emergency rooms that had been the standard source of care for the urban poor for decades already, Knowles wrote in 1969: "The long, hard bench with the four-hour wait, multiple referrals, incredible discontinuity of care and various other indignities suffered in an anti-social and decadent environment remains the order of the day in most ambulatory clinics in this country. A two-class system of care has prevailed whether it be the contrast between inpatient and outpatient care or private versus clinic patient" (1969, 178; quoted in Sardell 1988, 46).

These differences in access and quality of care in the United States reflect in part the nature of our class-biased health care delivery system. But what are we to make of class differences in health in countries with universal, free health care? Must we accept that these differences point to lifestyle and living environment alone?

Perhaps not. Italy also has universal free health care, but a study of the relationship between socioeconomic status and survival among AIDS patients (Perucci et al. 1999) found that even there, health care access and quality seem to be restricted for the poor. Examining survival rates of AIDS patients in the period 1993 to 1995, before the advent of effective antiretroviral therapy, researchers found no social class differences. In the period 1996 to 1997, however, after the introduction of such therapy, a marked social class difference in survival rates appeared. This in itself could be explained by class differences in adherence to treatment regimens; but the researchers took another step to pinpoint the problem. They looked at rates of survival for different treatment facilities, holding social class, sex, age, and cause of infection constant. If survival rates resulted from class-based patient behavior, there should have been no difference between facilities. In fact, there was a dramatic difference. Low-income patients fared much better at a metropolitan health center that served a predominantly middle-class population than at a low-income area clinic. It would appear that the quality of care at the two clinics itself was different, even in a country that seeks to provide equal access to the poor.

Environmentalism

The inaccessibility and poor quality of health care is, of course, only one of many social factors that can impair the health of the poor. We have already spent considerable time on the problems of social isolation and lack of access to knowledge, power, and wealth. These issues are dealt with more closely in the environmentalist works on poverty and health—a view that Sardell characterizes as "part of a long tradition of social medicine and . . . basic to the public health movement of mid-nineteenth-century America" (1988, 53). The environmentalist perspective is well summarized by the great health care reformer Michael M. Davis, in his 1918 work on dispensaries: "The community is becoming weary of a policy which spends two dollars a day for 'curing' a patient in a hospital and leaves untouched the home conditions which with reasonable certainty will compel the patient or his family to return for the same expensive process" (quoted in Sardell 1988, 41).

A good modern example of the environmentalist view is that of Lu Ann Aday (1993). In Aday's view, poor people—along with near poor single mothers, adolescents, people of color, the elderly, substance abusers, refugees, and those with chronic illnesses and mental health problems—are "differentially vulnerable to negative events," and they are therefore more likely to get sick and to stay sick than others, given a particular pathogen or stress. This elevated vulnerability is largely explained by three kinds of factors:

(a) *Social status*: The life circumstances that generally go with their social statuses carry high risks of exposure to stress and disease. They have less appropriate knowledge, and are less socially valued, and are physically weaker than others.

(b) *Social capital*: These people tend to have disrupted or weaker social networks and family ties, and to live in more-or-less isolated communities where effective voluntary help is hard to get.

(c) *Human capital*: Access to education, housing, health care, income, and employment is usually restricted for them.

Within the context of a society where appropriate compensation for these vulnerabilities is inadequate or unavailable, an illness or injury is likely to progress farther before being treated, to be treated less aggressively, and to be exacerbated by stress, poor nutrition and sanitation, lack of information, and exposure to additional risks. Aday pays particular attention to the health care system, which in most cases is not set up to treat the special problems of vulnerable populations at all, but instead offers uncoordinated, inadequate, spasmodic, and inappropriate interventions. As an antidote, she recommends a set of broad measures designed to redistribute opportunity more equally across social statuses, strengthen "non-mainstream" social networks (extended kin groups, co-residence units, voluntary associations, and so forth), and invest in community institutions that are able to provide appropriate human capital to these populations. Close cooperation will also be necessary among public agencies that provide the wide array of needed services.

Intervention Strategies

Given the difficulty of eliminating poverty- and social class-related differences in environment, behavior, and health access, all observers of the problem agree on the need for a stronger emphasis on preventing illness and maintaining wellness. Many writers point out that not only is the American health care system bogged down in a treatment-oriented approach at the expense of more efficient public health models, but what few preventive services are available are more accessible to the affluent than the poor. The question of who should pay for improved public health, however, contains a paradox: Sick people deserve help, and the healthy are often willing to pay (up to a point) for their treatment. But why should those with money—who after all are the healthier ones—pay to keep others healthy?

Attempts to deal with this question, even on a philosophical level, are rare; but Aday's (1993) work is one such attempt. Pointing out (much as I have tried to do in chapter 1) that our most important weapon against poverty and illness is compassion, and that compassion is a quality of families and communities, Aday sees the health of vulnerable populations as a matter for community action. Policy, she says, should support the efforts of communities to organize not only for more proactive and better integrated health services, but for greater social and economic equality and better access to the resources—education, housing, jobs, family and community supports—that reduce vulnerability. I agree. I return to this issue in chapters 7 and 8.

There is less agreement among reformers about exactly where the reform dollar can be most effectively spent. Those concerned with the effect of disability on income tend to emphasize (in addition to public health) occupational safety and accessibility of work for the partially disabled. Luft (1978), for example, suggests an array of measures that would include incentives for both employers and workers to reduce work hazards, greater attention to rehabilitation, incentives for hiring the partially disabled, and wage subsidies that would enable the health-impaired to work part-time or for lower wages. Adler et al., concerned as they are with the psychological and social effects of low income, suggest better training for health professionals in tailoring services to poor clients; and targeting low-income clients in health education efforts. They also point out that a more equal distribution of wealth would reduce stress for a larger population.

In my view, there is considerable value in each of these approaches to improving the health of the poor. Where all of these studies fall short is in failing to ask why our system persists in spite of its obvious inequality, ineffectiveness, and expense. What economic, political, and cultural forces support a type of health care that is at the same time the world's most expensive and one of its most unequal? Why does the nation fail to invest in the low-cost preventive strategies that would, in the opinion of many, go a long way toward closing the economic health gap? I will come back to this, but first let us look at the related question of responsibility.

Responsibility for the Health of the Poor

The German medical historian Henry Sigerist pointed out in the 1920s that our system of health care emerged from a number of deeply held cultural beliefs. Among these is the definition of illness in Western society as a misfortune that deserves sympathy and succor (Sigerist 1929). Accordingly, institutions for the treatment and care of the indigent sick and injured have always been part of the fabric of health care in Western societies. Before the development of modern technocratic states in the nineteenth century, this responsibility fell on families, communities, and beneficent functions of religious and guild organizations. In the American Colonies, almshouses brought together the homeless poor, orphans, the elderly, the insane, and the sick into family-like (and often squalid) care institutions. Alongside these in the larger cities there gradually developed, after 1750, larger public institutions, still supported by charity rather than taxes. In the nineteenth century, religious and ethnic hospitals began to develop as well, to serve particular sectors of society.

In the nineteenth century, many of the big public hospitals developed into prestigious medical teaching centers, featuring the now famous two-tiered care system of private rooms for the rich and public wards for the poor patients, the latter treated mainly as teaching cases. We have already commented above on the kind of care the poor received, but the directors of these hospitals were well aware that the two-tiered system was a financial necessity. When elite public hospitals for the rich were suggested, the directors would point out that the presence of the poor attracted charitable donations, and thereby kept the costs of the paying patients down (Starr 1982, 170).

After the Civil War, new developments in bacteriology began

to be used on a large scale to control epidemics, and this also resulted in public financing of some outpatient treatment of the poor with infectious diseases, and mass screenings of school children. Also in the nineteenth century, those city dwellers who were not sick enough to be in hospital, but could not afford a private physician (who would generally have treated them at home), were seen at charitably supported *dispensaries*, where apprentice doctors and medical students learned their trade (Rosenberg 1974). By the 1920s, however, the medical professions had grown powerful enough that they were generally able to prevent public authorities from doing more than identifying the infected and referring them to private physicians. The dispensaries had been absorbed into the teaching hospitals.

In the opening decades of the twentieth century, a movement for state-administered health insurance for workers was defeated by the combined efforts of private health insurance companies and state medical societies. In 1923, a federal bill that would have established public rural health centers to supplement the inadequate resources of rural doctors, was defeated by vehement lobbying efforts of the AMA. The AMA also categorically opposed, and virtually snuffed-out, contract medicine, by which low-income consumers founded fraternal societies and hired doctors on contract—a primitive form of health insurance (Sardell 1988; Starr 1982). The massive strides in science that made effective public health possible also led to the empowerment of a professional class that was vigorously hostile, not only toward public health, but to any participation whatsoever of the public sector in curative heath care. Between 1932 and 1950, advocates of federal universal health insurance tried three times to pass legislation guaranteeing access to health care for the American people—and each time they failed. It was not until the passage of Medicare and Medicaid in 1964 that major public responsibility for health became a fact; and to this day, these programs remain overwhelmingly curative and individualistic, almost ignoring the savings to be achieved through prevention and through community-based care.

We have seen that most modern academic experts on the health of the poor, regardless of their theory of causality, deplore the American emphasis on curative medicine at the expense of sanitation, education, and other more efficient preventive practices. Whether the ill health of the poor is largely a matter of environmental hazards, inadequate knowledge, lack of access to care, or emotional stress, prevention should work better than treatment, usually at a far lower cost—but we continue to flounder in the notion of a sacred, private, healing relationship.

The defeat of public responsibility for health has done much more than simply restrict the access of the poor to medical care. It has secured the private relationship between the individual patient and doctor as the terms of the discussion, almost eliminating both public health and social medicine from popular consciousness. In seeking to appease the private doctors, the public health authorities have promoted a kind of health education in which the individual is given near-absolute responsibility for his or her own health. The public is discouraged from even thinking about health as a community issue. Instead of public awareness of the health hazards of poverty and unregulated industry, the idea of the individual private checkup continues to be the standard of preventive health. The class-related health gap is in part an inevitable result.

It is within this context that the whole discussion of responsibility for the health of the poor takes place. It is a context in which it makes sense to conclude that the problem of ill health among the poor can be dealt with effectively by addressing personal characteristics like health knowledge and practices, lifestyle, stress, and access to individual care. Most advocates of better health for the poor place a large burden of responsibility on society—to provide a better environment, better health education, and better access to care. But by failing to question the existing arrangements of power within the health care industry, most academics end up merely repeating yet again the pleas of a century of social reformers.

Simply put, the emphasis on individualistic, curative medicine to the neglect of public health is the outcome of a profit-driven health care system. At first it was mainly the private physicians and hospitals that benefited from the private relationship of healers and patients. But once this equation was firmly established, there grew up around it and within it an enormous empire of wealth, represented by drug manufacturers and research labs, producers of medical equipment and supplies, insurance companies, the enormous government regulatory and university health science bureaucracies, the medical malpractice law industry, and specialized institutions such as nursing homes and psychiatric hospitals.

According to free market economic theory of course, this market-driven system should produce the highest quality results at the lowest cost. It is perplexing that its result is just the opposite, and many books have been written on why. Shameless greed and corruption is one well-documented reason; another is the control that wealth exerts over policy (see Sardell 1988, ch. 2). But both these causes are strengthened by our innocent passion for individual freedom. As long as the individual's right to choose remains the sacred totem of our health system, its results will always benefit the most competitive and acquisitive among us, at the expense of society in general, and the poor in particular.

Individuals can often improve their health by changing their habits. Communities can improve their residents' health by committing to a better environment and more equitable access to care. But if the health of the poor as a class is to change in a large and lasting way, one or more of the following things must happen: poverty must be reduced, or the health care of the poor must be made profitable, or health care must be freed from control by financial interests and opened to the operation of social values. To the extent that the ill health of the poor is an injustice, then, all social classes and all professions take part in the responsibility to address it. The role of the intellectual, it seems to me, is to clarify for society the nature of American health politics and culture.

Exercises And Study Questions

1.   Interview a low-income patient (or a health worker who is very familiar with such a patient) about a major illness of that patient. Try to understand how economics, environment, social and political attitudes, and the patient's own beliefs and behaviors have played into the illness, treatment, and outcome.

2.   The behaviorists point out that there is a continuous gradient in health from poor to rich. Can you think of any social or environmental hypotheses to explain this?

3. Visit for an hour or two one of the following: (a) an emergency room at a county hospital, (b) a welfare office, (c) a community clinic waiting room, (d) a waiting area (pharmacy, lab, and the like) of a large HMO. See how much you can find out about the health and health care of the people there.

4. Talk to some middle-class people with jobs unrelated to health care. Find out what they think about the health needs and resources of the poor in their community.

PART III

The Evolution and Role of Community Health Centers

T hroughout this book, I have been presenting the ill health of the poor as a problem—something to be diagnosed, explained, and combated by the concerned health care worker. That approach necessarily draws a gloomy picture of our health care system, our society, and even our species. In this chapter and the next, I present the hopeful side of working with the poor as a health professional. I show some of the things that have been accomplished, and ask how these accomplishments can be learned from and built upon.

I begin by focusing on the nation's Community Health Centers (CHCs), a program created by the Johnson administration's Office of Economic Opportunity (OEO) in 1965 as part of the War on Poverty legislation. In singling out CHCs, I have to apologize for slighting the hundreds of other nonprofit and volunteer health programs for the poor that have made and are making a difference in cities and towns all over America. I have selected CHCs for four reasons:

- First, the CHC movement as a whole is big and visible. As such, information about it is easy to obtain.
- Second, CHCs represent an unusual success in building a structure for the health care of the poor. Although most centers are now being battered by a host of financial problems stemming from profit-driven health care reform, their remaining strength, and the good they have already accomplished, deserves understanding if progress is to be made.
- Third, the idea behind the CHC movement—linking health with the other needs and institutions of communities, and giving consumers a voice in their own care—while not unique or new, strikes me as a promising one.
- Fourth, as a board member of a CHC for six years, I have some experience in how the concept works at the community level.

What Is a Community Health Center?

Although there are many kinds of clinics serving the needs of low-income populations throughout the country, I will use the term Community Health Center to refer to

- a nonprofit corporation serving a defined local community or migrant worker population;
- delivering a variety of services including primary health care;
- with a board of directors drawn from its users and other community residents;
- dedicated by charter to the goal of providing the best possible quality health care, at maximum efficiency, to the most economically disadvantaged members of the community;
- receiving support largely from public sources for health care to the poor.

As of 1995, the National Association of Community Health Centers listed 822 such CHCs in the United States, operating a total of 2,200 health care delivery sites, serving 8.8 million patients with 31 million visits annually, and managing a total of $2.1 billion in transactions (NACHC 1996).

Since the clients at these clinics are overwhelmingly poor, the CHCs obviously could not function without massive public support. Most CHCs receive funding (average 35 percent of budget) from Public Health Service Act Grants for health centers (section 330), migrant workers (section 329), and the homeless (section 340). As so-called Federally Qualified Health Centers (FQHCs), providing a list of basic services to predominantly low-income clientele, most also receive support (average 33 percent of budget) from Medicaid *reasonable cost* reimbursement. Other sources include state and local funds for indigent care (average 11 percent of budget), patient payments (7 percent), health insurance (8 percent), and Medicare (5 percent) (NACHC 1996). The mix of payers differs considerably from community to community and location to location, depending on the kind of services offered and the kind of clientele in the area. For example, the Over 60 Health Center in Berkeley, California, serving the low-income elderly in Alameda County, receives about 45 percent of its reimbursement income from Medicare and Medicaid payments.

The emphasis on local control results in a huge variety with regard to the specific missions of the CHCs and the details of their ownership, administration, financing, and relationships with their communities—a variety impossible to characterize here. There are CHCs that serve primarily homeless, or immigrants, or Spanish speaking, or elderly. There are those specializing in detoxification and rehabilitation, or urgent care, or perinatal care, or assisted living for the frail and disabled. There are those that form partnerships with local hospitals, or physicians' groups, or health departments, or universities, or housing services. The range of approaches to local conditions shows astounding creativity.

Evolution of the CHCs

The 1950s and early 1960s was a period of economic growth, rising living standards, and optimism in America. It was one of those periods, like the end of the nineteenth century, when science, government, and technology seemed to be coming up with solutions, one by one, to all of humanity's problems. As such, it was also a time when those left out of the general prosperity—people of color, the aged, the poor—felt their plight all the more keenly, and began demanding to be heard. Mainstream America, lulled into euphoria by prosperity, was jolted awake and discovered poverty.

Working with a strongly Democratic congress, the liberal Johnson administration faced a growing storm of civil rights demonstrations and riots beginning in 1963. The time was right for synergy between the voices of the marginalized and those of reformers in Washington, who seemed confident that inequality in America could be reduced. Johnson called this agenda The Great Society; and in 1963 initiated its centerpiece, the War on Poverty. The liberal view of health care was that it was too centralized and hospital based, and that it was failing to serve the needs of the poor, the elderly, and the mentally ill. The solution was to put a greater emphasis on prevention, on outpatient services, and on the involvement of communities—the core principles of the CHCs.

Although government sponsorship of community clinics serving the poor was a new development in America, the idea of such clinics was by no means new here; local attempts to establish privately financed clinics for the poor reach back at least to the early 1900s. But lacking a public mandate, such attempts were always short-lived. Local physicians, fearing a loss of income if low-cost services opened in their community, closed ranks and stifled each attempt. The Cincinnati Social Unit, opened by wealthy philanthropists in 1918, drew national attention but closed in 1920 under pressure from the medical community. In the 1920s, the noted sociologist and social reformer Michael M. Davis propounded the idea of *health centers*, which would employ salaried physicians and coordinate the efforts of public health authorities and private philanthropic organizations to provide comprehensive services to the poor. Several attempts were made to implement this model, notably the Cornell Clinic, but it, too was opposed by the medical establishment and soon died (Sardell 1988, 39–42).

The so-called group practice movement, another attempt at improving health access of the less affluent, began in the 1930s. In 1932 the prestigious private research group, the Committee on the Costs of Medical Care (CCMC), issued a high-profile report in which it supported the idea of group practice—a kind of private health co-op under which groups of consumers contract with physicians for their care. The CCMC apparently had not studied the political implications of this recommendation, however, and attempts to implement it were systematically suppressed by medical societies. Group practices set up in Elk City, Oklahoma, and in Los Angeles drew national attention, but could not survive against AMA boycotts. In one famous 1943 case, the American Medical Association was successfully sued for violation of antitrust laws, but was never prosecuted and the incident blew over (Sardell 1988, 44; Starr 1982, 261–263).

Even given the liberal political climate of the 1960s, then, it is surprising that federal support for community clinics succeeded. Not only was the community clinic legislation a challenge to the absolute autonomy of the medical profession—as the group practice movement had been, it also sought to change the way health care was planned and organized. Private practice was (and still is)

(a) overwhelmingly centered on the individual doctor-patient relationship;

(b) curative rather than preventive;

(c) based on a referral system that divides the patient's needs among a host of uncoordinated specialties;

(d) blind to the social and environmental context of care; and

(e) planned and organized largely by, and for, medical professionals.

The Clinics, by contrast, were to

(a) provide preventive services;

(b) offer comprehensive care;

(c) tailor services to local conditions;

(d) be guided by autonomous lay boards;

(e) be low in cost and open to everyone who wanted them.

How, then, did the CHCs get a foothold in the American health care system? The AMA did in fact oppose the initial idea; but in addition to the intense pressure for reform brought by the civil rights movement, there appear to have been several factors that contributed to its success. One was the political role played by the plight of the elderly. The low-income elderly are generally looked upon as deserving poor, and their medical needs as especially worthy of attention. Since the mid-1950s, pressure had been growing in congress for federal health legislation to ease their suffering, and the CHC movement was tied in to this trend.

Another factor was that the liberals of the 1960s promoted the idea that attempts to relieve poverty required experimentation with new solutions; and the CHCs were first presented not as a new institution, but as a small, self-limiting experiment—a demonstration project, located in the president's office and not part of any ongoing bureaucracy. To co-opt resistance from organized medicine, the first grants for demonstration clinics went to hospitals and medical schools; and the point was made that the goal was not to reduce the costs of medicine for the majority, but to give access to a group of clients who currently had none (Sardell 1988).

Under Sargent Shriver, director of the new OEO, were a number of energetic and effective liberals. Julius Richmond, director of the Head Start program and assistant director of OEO, was a pediatrician who recognized the importance of health care in the War on Poverty. Together with Shriver and psychiatrist Joseph English, he decided to establish the Office of Health Affairs of the OEO in 1965. They recruited Elizabeth Bamberger Shorr and Sanford Kravitz to work on the development of models for the community clinic idea, who in return recruited Count Gibson, chair of the Department of Preventive Medicine at Tufts, and H. Jack Geiger. Gibson and Geiger were given a million dollars to plan and initiate the first CHCs—one at a housing project in Columbia Point in Boston, and one in Mileston in rural Holmes County, Mississippi. They envisioned that control of the CHCs should be mainly in the hands of the users, knowing full well that this spelled conflict with the medical establishment. But they brought the prestige of Tufts University to their side of the conflict (Couto 1991, 267–275). Shorr, English, and others at the Office of Health Affairs adopted a new style of administration, often getting to know the recipients of OHA grants personally, and serving as advocates for them within the Washington bureaucratic culture.

Still another factor was the role of the U.S. Public Health Service. Thanks to its historical role in monitoring health statistics, promoting health, and controlling epidemics, the USPHS had a long-standing interest in the health of the poor. During the 1960s, particularly, many liberal physicians joined the USPHS as a way of participating in the new liberal atmosphere, or as an alternative to serving in the Vietnam War. In 1966, Congress passed the Comprehensive Health Planning and Public Health Services Act, which in section 314 (e) authorized the USPHS to fund projects on a regional basis that would improve the integration of health services. The reform-minded officials at USPHS decided to use this money to fund community clinics, and between 1966 and 1972, they funded fifty-five centers serving 850,000 people (Sardell 1988, 72–73). A constituency for the clinics was taking shape.

At the community level, there was often synergy between the CHC movement and the civil rights movement. In 1969, for example, a group of medical students at Vanderbilt University wanted to work for civil rights in the poor, predominantly black communities of western Tennessee and the predominantly white towns of eastern Kentucky. They established the Student Health Coalition, an organization that sent medical and other university students into poor communities to help raise consciousness around health and economic issues. Among the many excellent results of the Student Health Coalition in the 1970s was the founding of community clinics in many Appalachian and western Tennessee towns (Couto 1982). Couto also documents the founding of community clinics in rural Arkansas, Alabama, and Georgia's Sea Islands in the late 1960s and early 1970s. Once rural blacks had begun to question the Southern white establishment, the health needs of their communities often led them to establish clinics (Couto 1991).

The relationship between the government, the medical establishment, local power structures, and the clinic projects was often far from smooth, however. Given their different cultures, serious conflict was inevitable. Community boards often had different priorities, and different ideas about cost effectiveness, than physicians or bureaucrats. The physicians often insisted on prioritizing the quality of health care; while local activists often sought other ways of empowering their communities to take charge of their own affairs, such as teaching literacy and political participation. At times the tension in meetings would get so high that participants feared violence (Couto 1991, 280). The fact that this gripping and inspiring story of courage, dedication, and conflict over the health rights of poor communities is not better known tells us a great deal about the priorities of America's mainstream media and education system.

By the early 1970s, however, the CHCs had already developed bases of support in many communities, and within the federal agencies that funded them. This support, along with liberal leadership in congress, served to sustain the movement during the attacks of the Nixon and Ford administrations. Nixon tried to dismantle the War on Poverty, in the process transferring the CHCs from OEO to the Department of Health, Education and Welfare (DHEW), over which he then sought to exert strong conservative control. But the centers survived in spite of this, banding together in 1971 to form the National Association of Community Health Centers (NACHC), the political voice of the movement informally referred to as *Nack*. With the help of strong pro-center voices such as Senator Edward Kennedy and Congressman Paul Rogers, Congress passed separate funding for the CHCs over President Ford's veto in 1975. At the same time, the new administrative home of the centers at DHEW, known as the Bureau of Community Health Services (BCHS), developed a plan called the Rural Health Initiative, to put more funds into the development of health centers in the most underserved rural areas. This plan proved to be a popular one because a relatively small investment could produce dramatic results in many of the recipient communities.

The Carter administration (1977–1981) was generally favorable to the CHC movement, but the centers continued to have problems. They were expected to provide comprehensive primary care to their clients, but were often unable to get reimbursed for many services, such as transportation and social counseling, that are essential if the poor are to have access. An estimated one-half to two-thirds of people living below the poverty line in 1978 did not qualify for Medicaid; and a majority of the states would not reimburse CHCs for treating Medicaid patients anyway. That year, there were 574 CHCs nationally, but they were only serving about 10 percent of the country's poor and underserved population, and many were not able to offer comprehensive services.

In his studies of community clinics in eastern Kentucky and western Tennessee, Couto saw that many poor communities were energized by the idea of building and running their own clinic to fill an obvious shortage of health care. This enthusiasm brought forth generous volunteer help and donations. People with little education or administrative experience learned to assemble and run complex organizations, and to sell their mission to health professionals and local bureaucrats, an empowering experience. But once the centers had been built and federal funding secured, the problem of sustaining them often proved overwhelming. The funding agencies' dual requirements that the clinics (a) be self-sustaining, and (b) serve the poorest in their communities, was self-defeating. Couto quotes a health council member from White Oak, Tennessee:

Let's say the way it works here, through this area, if we come up with 50 percent of what we spend, we'd be doing good. That's the way I feel about it. That is, if you're going to doctor the people they [DHEW] require you to doctor. That's the people I'm interested in first, you know . . . the people who can't pay. You see, the thing they tell you is that you've got to make dollar for dollar, and then they turn right around and tell you you've got to doctor people who can't pay—maybe half that many.

Well, alright. It's like putting legs on a table, and cutting one of them off. You know if you saw it off, it's going to fall over. Well, how're you going to doctor the people that can't pay you, and then pay your bills? (Couto 1982, 81–82)

While the urban clinics shared many of the financial problems of their rural colleagues, the latter had special difficulties. One was the absolute shortage of money throughout their service area, while urban clinics could often turn to wealthy benefactors in the same city. Another rural disadvantage was the relative scarcity of both medical professionals and potential lay leaders to serve the clinics, and this problem was exacerbated by the necessity of securing government funds. As Couto explains, bureaucrats tend to adhere rigidly to uniform regulations that might be quite inappropriate in a given community. They also tend to put authority in the hands of professionals, however ill-informed about or marginal to the community—rather than laymen, however experienced and trusted in local society. Under these conditions local lay leadership tends to burn out rather quickly, and the enthusiasm and commitment of the community cannot be sustained without it. Some rural clinics have failed as a result of these combined difficulties. The irony is that some of the failures were probably unnecessary, if the health services bureaucracy had been more flexible about reimbursement and adherence to regulations. The general trend since the 1970s, however, has been less flexibility, not more.

Communities both rural and urban, fortunate enough to have health centers, almost always seek ways to keep them operating even under stressful conditions—usually through generous private donations and volunteer help. Local politicians often find the clinics popular among average voters, and seek to liberalize state and local policies affecting them. This grassroots popularity of the clinics has, I believe, kept most of them alive during the present conservative era, which began in earnest under President Reagan.

The Reagan administration moved swiftly to eliminate federal support for CHCs. The BCHS was reshuffled and downsized, promoting people who either had no appropriate experience, or were known to be hostile to the program. An attempt was made to shunt federal support to the states, in the form of block grants, and in 1982, Reagan cut CHC funds by 24 percent. Other cuts, in maternal and child health (18 percent), preventive programs (37.5 percent), and alcohol and drug treatment (24 percent) likewise hurt the programs of many CHCs. The result was a vigorous political fight in congress, during which most cuts were eventually restored. But the liberals could not keep the CHC budget in pace with inflation, so that between 1981 and 1986, there was an overall 20 percent decline in real federal funding (Sardell 1988, 195).

The battle in Washington over the clinics' budget does not tell the whole story of their struggle to survive in an increasingly restrictive political climate. Some regional BCHS personnel and other officials responsible for the management of federal support took the view that clinic management continuously had to prove their honesty and effectiveness in order to continue receiving funds. For many, the increased amount of time spent on paperwork, and increased delays in securing grants and reimbursement were added to an already precarious financial situation.

In the 1994 elections, Republicans achieved a majority in both the House and the Senate, reversing a forty-year Democratic edge in congress. In 1996, congress passed the Personal Responsibility and Work Opportunity Reconciliation Act, which represents a dramatic reduction in the federal government's responsibility for the problems of the poor. I have dealt at some length in chapter 5 with the conservative view of poverty and welfare, and the effects of this view on health and on community clinics. As I write this in 1999, it is too early to see what long-term impact this latest political trend will have on the CHC movement, but the implications are serious. It is likely that

- the number of low-income Americans without health insurance will grow, forcing CHCs to rely more on private charity or to limit access;
- welfare payments will be smaller for more people, leaving them less cash for noncovered health needs, and for healthy housing and nutrition;
- the average CHC client will be sicker when seen, requiring more expensive care;
- state and local health care payments to low-income patients will be smaller and will cover fewer services;
- large HMOs will garner a larger share of insured and low-risk patients, leaving CHCs and emergency rooms with a larger proportion of the uninsured and chronically ill;
- administrative costs of community clinics will increase substantially, lowering their efficiency.

When the CHC movement began, many of its architects viewed it as a test model for the development of an entirely new way of delivering health care in the United States, a system for the poor and nonpoor alike. Its emphasis on prevention and primary care promised greater efficiency; its dedication to accessibility and local accountability promised greater justice and higher quality. A number of studies indicate that some CHCs, at least, have succeeded in fulfilling this vision, even under the harsh political climate I have described. CHCs tend to have lower costs and lower hospitalization rates per user than hospital outpatient departments, regardless of the users' socioeconomic status (Freeman et al. 1982). One study compared counties with CHCs against those without, and found systematically lower infant mortality rates for all races in the former (Sardell 1988, 229–230). Another found that regular CHC use results in a 33 percent average savings to Medicaid for nonmaternity cases, and a 10–14 percent savings overall, while at the same time CHC users received equal or better care than those using other outpatient services on twenty-one quality measures (Starfield et al. 1994).

The Over 60 Health Center: History of a CHC

There is so much diversity in the nation's CHCs that the history of a single clinic cannot hope to capture the details of the movement. Geographic region, urban versus rural location, size, ethnic makeup, the type and range of services and funding sources—these are just some of the major sources of variation. But in this chapter I want to convey a concrete sense of the process by which the clinics have evolved and functioned, and that goal can be brought closer by recounting an actual example. I will use the Over 60 Health Center in Berkeley, California as my example, for the simple reason that my wife Else and I have been involved with Over 60, in one way or another, for most of its history. Else served on the Board from 1984 until 1993, and I have from 1994 to the present. In telling the story of Over 60, I will focus on the actors as much as possible, since I have already given some of the broad political background. I am much indebted in what follows to Judith Turiel, who shared excerpts of interviews she did with several of the key actors in 1991–1992.

Lillian Rabinowitz is an outgoing person who smiles and laughs easily. When she speaks, she seems to choose her words carefully, in an effort to make herself as clear as possible. This might be a habit she developed during her two careers, first as a social worker, and later as a primary school teacher. Lillian was an energetic sixty-two-year old when she met Gray Panthers founder Maggie Kuhn in 1973—a meeting that led her that same year to help found a chapter of the elders' rights organization in Berkeley.

One of the first things the Gray Panthers chapter did was to begin the work of founding a free clinic for the low-income elderly in the area. Lillian had retired from her teaching job two years earlier, and her oldest child had recently left home. She and her colleagues on the Gray Panthers board were aware that many older people in the area were living in nursing homes, under less than ideal conditions. Lillian, who had been to England and learned about the superior system of geriatric care there, believed that many of these elders would be living better lives at home, if they had had access to more appropriate health care earlier. In February of 1974, she and her colleagues applied to the the City of Berkeley for a CETA grant to study community needs for long-term care, and in the fall of that year received the grant.

The need was clear. No one in the East Bay was providing comprehensive health services to the elderly population. Especially vulnerable were low-income elderly, whose insurance—if any—rarely covered the services of a doctor who was trained in geriatrics. In 1975 the Berkeley Gray Panthers applied for a forty thousand dollar grant from the Oakland Area Agency on Aging, an Older Americans Act Title III agency, to start a center "to provide comprehensive integrated health services for older residents of Berkeley, Albany, North Oakland, and Emeryville." The program was not to compete with existing medical services, but was to provide health screening, health education, referral services, crisis intervention, and outpatient supportive services, relying heavily on volunteers, working out of donated space. Some county revenue-sharing funds were also made available.

The grant was awarded in April of 1975, and the search for an administrative home began. Their first effort was to find an existing clinic that could add the service, but after looking at the available services, they were discouraged. "But we decided it wouldn't work out well. If frail old people had to go to a clinic where people were freaked out [on drugs] it would scare the bejeezus out of them. . . . The Black Panther clinic targeted only the Black Community, and the Women's Health Collective didn't take men" (Rabinowitz, quoted in Turiel, 1995, 5).

In July of that year, the Gray Panthers finally worked out an agreement with the Berkeley City Health Department to administer the project, but with the stipulation that only those elderly with incomes below the poverty line would be eligible to participate. Disappointed, they decided to accept the terms, meanwhile organizing to remove the income test and make the services free to everyone who applied. A series of skirmishes with the county attorney ensued, but the issue was not resolved.

On January 15, 1976, the Geriatric Health Services Program opened its doors in a rented storefront at the corner of San Pablo Avenue and Russell Street in Berkeley. Paid staff included a geriatric nurse practitioner who doubled as administrator, a receptionist, a janitor, a secretary, and a community health worker. Other service personnel volunteered—some twenty-five in all, including nurses, social workers, secretaries, and University of California students in social work, health care administration, and psychology. Another cadre of volunteers designed, printed, and distributed fliers, wrote news releases, carried out statistical studies of the community, and helped the clients in a variety of ways.

In the beginning, according to the early participants, the free services of the clinic were by today's standards lavish. "You felt like you were welcome," as Leatha Phillips says. A brochure from the period describes the services:

> On the first visit, clinic staff nurses and physician collect background information, take a health history, record both prescription and non-prescription medications taken, review food and diet patterns, record height and weight, ascertain problem areas in mobility and activities of daily living, take pulse and blood pressure readings, and give tests for vision, hearing, and urine.
>
> From there, the client will spend an hour or more completing the exam with the nurse who reviews background data, examines ears, mouth, skin, feet, and other areas; takes a tonometer reading for glaucoma; makes an assessment; then discusses problem areas and plans with the client.
>
> If no problem areas are identified and the client is found to be in good health, the nurse may make recommendations for health maintenance. The client is encouraged to return at six-month intervals to monitor changes in health status.

If problem areas are identified, the nurse provides follow-up counseling and treatment, and, where appropriate, referrals. In fact, a log for the second week of January, 1978, shows that the clinic's three nurses saw fifty-nine clients, and spent an average of fifty-six minutes with each.

But it did not prove easy to convince people that free services like this were really a good idea, especially since the clinic had at first asked for income data from clients. Moreover, people wanted first and foremost to see a doctor, and when it first opened physicians were only available intermittently, on a volunteer basis. In the early years, then, acceptance was slow. The founders were a racially mixed group, but most were outsiders, not known in the neighborhood. One of them, Charlotte Knight, who was white, used to canvas the neighborhood together with Sylvia Brown, the community health worker paid by the City of Berkeley, who is black. Twenty years later Charlotte reminisced: "We walked the streets with clinic flyers. . . . She was a black lady, hip to black people. . . . The clinic didn't have enough clients. People weren't coming in. It was a great struggle to be accepted. You know, there were people who opposed all these old white ladies coming in and founding a clinic right there in the heart of the black community" (Turiel 1992, 6). Charlotte died in 1999.

By January 1978, the clinic had seen approximately a thousand clients, and had an annual operating budget of about sixty-four thousand dollars. Sources of income included property tax General Funds and Revenue Sharing Funds from the County of Alameda, support from the City of Berkeley Health Department, foundation grants, and private donations. Leatha Phillips, a black neighbor who ran a restaurant called the Bus Stop next door to the site, donated her space and time for fund-raisers, and after a day's work also walked the neighborhood, knocking on doors to tell people about the service. A small, grand motherly woman with a strong physique, Mrs. Phillips was on the board of Over 60, and working to promote the clinic throughout South Berkeley until her death in 1998, at the age of eighty-one. "I've held every position on the Board," she told me, "except president. I wouldn't let them put me president." She remembered nostalgically the many potlucks, raffles, and neighborhood fund-raisers of the early clinic.

"People will give to something like that. You'd be surprised. Even if it's only five dollars, even if they don't have anything, they're glad to do it."

In the wake of Proposition 13, which severely reduced the local tax base, Berkeley city officials declared that the city could no longer take administrative responsibility for Over 60. Accordingly, in 1978 the clinic was incorporated as an independent nonprofit corporation, the Over 60 Health Clinic, and joined the Alameda Health Consortium, a group of nine primary care clinics serving primarily low-income clients throughout the county. The era of tax revolt had begun in California, and for the community clinics, it meant a strenuous battle to survive. That year, Proposition 13, the property tax reform bill, went into effect, as a direct result of which Over 60 lost more than a third of their budget. In the 1980 election, another ballot initiative—Proposition 9, this one aimed to cut state income taxes by 50 percent—further jeopardized services to the poor in California. The state threatened to cut $400 million from its Medicaid budget in 1982.

But somehow, Over 60 continued to grow. In 1982, the assistant director, Marty Lynch, became director. Marty, trained in counseling psychology, had held a number of administrative positions with community health and social service projects in the area. An outgoing and personable young administrator, Marty had already built a wide network of friends among other administrators in local government and health care. His contacts with city and county officials, local doctors and hospital administrators, and even state level politicians, were personal and cordial—a skill that has proved invaluable to Over 60 throughout the past seventeen years.

The year Marty Lynch became director, a physician was also hired as medical director—Dr. Kathryn Borgenicht, newly certified in internal medicine. This meant Over 60 could provide complete primary care services, and could bill Medicare, which they began to do in January of 1983. But the site at San Pablo Avenue and Russel Street had already become too small for the increased work and clientele, and the clinic had to move.

Nineteen eighty-three was a dramatic year for the clinic. Funds had been raised to purchase new space, and a 4,600–square-foot site—a former post office—was found at 1860 Alcatraz, about three miles from the original site, but still in the predominantly low-income African American area of south Berkeley. Thanks to the new site, dental services were procured for the first time, through the National Health Services Corps. Added revenues from Medicare and Medicaid, plus a Primary Care Grant from the state, doubled their budget between 1982 and 1984—to four hundred and eighty-nine thousand dollars.

At the same time, the antiwelfare policies of the Reagan administration began to be felt. In order to be eligible for the NHSC services, Over 60 was required to conform to the *self-sufficiency rule*, and to begin charging clients for services on a sliding scale. Alameda County quickly followed suit with the same demand of its publicly supported clinics. Several local agencies serving the poor already had been forced to close, but with the help of grants from the liberal Berkeley city government, Over 60 survived.

Almost every year throughout the 1980s, the clinic added new services, and as a result new sources of funding. In 1982 it was primary care and outreach to the homebound, and 1983, dental care. In 1985, they added mental health services, in 1986 case management, hospital coverage, and twenty-four-hour call service. In 1988 and 1989, they added services for the homeless elderly and management of Alzheimer's patients. The same year a licensed podiatrist was hired, to provide foot care services which had been provided by the nurses until then. In addition to city, county, and state grants, the clinic had gotten support from the Koret Foundation, the Cowell Foundation, the Haas Fund, the King's Daughters, the Kaiser Family Foundation, Blue Cross, the Robert Wood Johnson Foundation, the Irvine Family Fund, and the American Cancer Society. The 1989 budget was a million dollars.

Reimbursement by Medicare and Medicaid, and skill at grant writing, provided a degree of stability to Over 60's chronically shaky finances. In 1991, Over 60 was certified as a Federally Qualified Health Center (FQHC). This meant that as a community-owned nonprofit clinic providing primary care services to a predominantly poor population, they were entitled to be reimbursed at *reasonable cost* by Medicare and Medicaid, rather than accepting the usual below-cost rates. But throughout the 1990s, maintaining public support has continued to present a serious problem. California counties are responsible for administering many services to the poor, but their financing comes largely from the state, where they have little political voice. Always short of money for services, county budget hearings annually become the scenes of intense lobbying by local clinics and other agencies—and most come away with less than they need to provide quality services to their entire potential clientele.

With the failure of the Clinton administration's attempt to overhaul health care financing in 1993–1994, the situation did not improve for community clinics. The thirty-year "crisis" of exploding health care costs had reached a point where the so-called payers—government, private insurance companies and HMOs, and employers—could reasonably demand that providers should get less money, while continuing to meet the demand for services.[1] I have dealt with the general effects of the supposed solution, namely Managed Care, in chapter 6.[2] Let us look more closely at the impact on Over 60.

In the late 80s and early 90s, the payers—insurance companies, Medicaid, and Medicare—began to experiment with managed care contracts. This is a strategy, you will recall, whereby the payer gets providers to bid against each other for contracts to provide services to the payer's clients. The aim, of course, is to reduce the costs of the insurer, by ultimately paying less and getting the same services. (Let us note the all-important but unanswerable question: Is cheap health care ever the same as expensive health care, even in a strictly clinical sense?) Providers in Over 60's region accordingly began to join the bidding process. The payers accept a given fee as primary providers to a given patient or group of patients, and then contract with providers to deliver the actual care. The risk of being able to give the contracted services for less money than the premium is first accepted by the payer, and then passed on to the provider.

In order to make this risk contracting work, it is necessary for both the insurer and the provider to have a high volume of business. This allows them to enroll relatively healthy patients as well as relatively sick ones, in the hope of achieving an actual average cost per patient that falls within the premium.

Accordingly, both payers and providers (sometimes, as in the case of the large hospitals, the same entity) began to advertise aggressively to recruit insured patients. Since older people have Medicare (and many of the poorer ones have Medicaid as well), the elderly population of Over 60s catchment area became the target of vigorous recruitment campaigns. The large, well-capitalized payers began to send speakers to every senior center, subsidized housing project, and lunch program in the East Bay, to sell their product—a list of services available through their own providers. The sales reps handed out stacks of attractive, glossy brochures, hired well-trained speakers armed with dazzling slides and videos— and paid for a sumptuous lunch. In many cases, they also offered comprehensive care at very low premiums—typically for no premium at all if the patient was covered by Medicare Parts A and B—a strategy called Zero Premium Medicare.

This practice suddenly meant that Over 60 was at a serious competitive disadvantage, for several reasons. First, Over 60 serves an overwhelmingly poor clientele of predominantly frail elderly— in other words the sickest and most costly kinds of patients to care for. The risk of treating this group is therefore far higher than that of younger or more affluent elderly groups. Over 60 would either have to negotiate higher per capita rates than other providers, or recruit another type of patient, or be driven out of business by larger, better capitalized organizations.

Second, Over 60, as a community-owned service, is committed to the mission of providing better services to its users than they could get from a private or for-profit source. This is no mere platitude. The Board consistently makes decisions on the basis of their effects on patient care, often at the cost of so-called efficiency. Giving better service tends to cost more money, even when it is done by idealistic people who are willing to work for less pay.

Third, in order to fulfill this mission, the clinic not only has to raise money through grants and donations, it also has to charge patients on a sliding scale for services not covered by their insurance. Some of its low-income clientele were now forced to choose between Over 60 and something cheaper.

Fourth, the competition for managed care contracts obviously rewards large organizations with a high volume of patients and a large budget—organizations that can spread losses, buy technology, impress clients and politicians, and intimidate competitors. This is why the emergence of managed care has been accompanied by a frenzy of mergers throughout the health care industry. But Over 60 is not only small, it is a specialty clinic, designed and destined to stay small. Its charter is not to serve everyone in its vicinity, nor even all the poor. While the clinic can and does collaborate with other CHCs and other health organizations as a semiautonomous member of a team, as a low-income geriatric clinic, with an array of services and staff abilities specifically designed to serve the poor and frail elderly, Over 60 could not easily merge with other providers without the serious danger of losing its mission.

In order to keep its patients, then, Over 60 and other CHCs had to negotiate contracts with the larger payers—Prudential, Kaiser, Aetna, Pacificare, and Healthnet. Patients could then sign up with one of these plans, and use Over 60 as their provider. Nor was this a happy solution to the new problem. It amounted to a drain on Over 60s already strained resources, in several ways:

- It involved the administrative staff in a time-consuming task that did not directly produce improved operations. In addition to contracting with new payers, most of the insurance plans brought together networks of providers—hospitals, practice groups, HMOs, consortia—and relationships with other providers in a given plan also had to be worked out.
- It required that Over 60 invest directly in marketing their services, not just to enroll new patients, but also to keep the very people they were already serving. Surveys of patient satisfaction were needed, in order to correct perceived deficiencies in service. Mailing lists had to be compiled, brochures and newsletters printed
- Staff had to be familiar with many more kinds of payment schemes, and spent a good deal more time on paperwork. Patients were often confused about what their plans would pay for, and extra time had to be spent advising them.
- Managed care contracting required the keeping of detailed records on such things as actual and average costs per visit

and per patient, the productivity (rate of patients seen) of each provider, and the constantly shifting numbers of patients covered by each type of insurance. This meant the overhauling of the clinic's computing and filing systems.

- Many of the managed care plans did not cover the services Over 60 found most helpful to the low-income frail elderly, such as home visits, case management, social services, transportation, and mental health. The clinic had to continue to find other ways to pay for these.

On the plus side, as of 1999, Over 60 still maintains its status as a Federally Qualified Health Center (FQHC), and therefore is still able to collect reasonable costs for services covered by Medicare and Medicaid. The Clinton administration has announced plans to phase out the FQHC provision over the next five years, however—a move that may close many CHCs.

Meanwhile, Over 60 had outgrown its facility at 1860 Alcatraz. The administrative offices had been moved to rented space at 1840, a few doors west, and a new site was opened at a senior center on Edes Avenue in east Oakland; but there was still a shortage of space for the main clinics. Some years earlier, the board had purchased a large lot at the corner of Sacramento and Alcatraz; and began to explore the possibility of building a new clinic there. A project for a combined clinic and low-income housing site was approved by the board in 1994; and in 2000, Over 60 opened a new 17,000–square-foot clinic at the site. The clinic is jointly owned and occupied by Over 60 and the Center for Elders Independence, another nonprofit serving disabled elders in the neighborhood. In the same building, above the clinic, a low-income housing developer, Resources for Community Development (RCD) built and operates forty units of HUD-financed housing. The total project cost $10 million.

In 1993, the State of California had announced its intention to begin a demonstration project in which Medicaid would be paid through managed care contracts in eleven counties, including Alameda, where Over 60 resides. There would be two Medicaid providers in each county (one public and one private) and certain categories of local Medicaid clients (about half the total Medicaid population of 276,000 users) would be required to sign up with one of these. Over the next three years the Alameda county health care industry evolved its two organizations, one managed by Blue Cross, the other by a coalition of public facilities and CHCs called the Alameda Alliance for Health, of which Over 60 is a member. It was clear from the outset that this was meant as a cost-reduction measure, and that Medicaid reimbursement rates were due to diminish. The question was, how much.

Greater provider risk, and therefore the need for greater efficiency and greater volume, was now extended to this gigantic new group of patients. Soon after Medicaid contracting was announced, Over 60 was approached by another CHC, the Berkeley Primary Care Access Clinic (BPCAC), to explore the possibility of a merger. BPCAC had been created in 1991, to provide primary and urgent care to the predominantly low-income clientele that had formerly used the emergency facilities at Herrick Hospital. Most of their business consisted of perinatal and pediatric services to Medicaid and uninsured low-income families, and primary and urgent care to Berkeley's indigent and homeless population. They were also financially stressed, for most of the same reasons that Over 60 was. About half their visits—some eight thousand annually—had Medicaid coverage. A merger was considered as a way of increasing the size and diversity of the two operations, thereby improving both their positions in managed care contracting.

In 1995, Over 60 took over another troubled community clinic—West Berkeley Family Practice—and in July 1996, they merged with BPCAC. The three clinics, now known collectively as Lifelong Medical Care, had a combined total of ninety-five thousand patients, seen for a total of thirty-three thousand visits per year. The annual budget was about $5.5 million.

So far, Over 60 and its sister clinics have survived the shift to managed care fairly well. About 14 percent of their total patient visits are paid under capitated plans—either Medicaid or Medicare. The Alameda Alliance for Health, of which Over 60 and BPCAC are members, had recruited about 80 percent of the 112,000 mandated Medicaid managed care population who had chosen a primary care provider as of mid-1997.

However, the clinics continue to be battered by financial problems. In November 1997, cuts in Medicaid reimbursement rates and in county support for indigent care forced the clinics for the first time to stop accepting new uninsured patients. Several patient requests per day began to be referred to the county hospital emergency room for the first time in the clinics' history, until a weekly volunteer clinic opened in February 1999. BPCAC has also had to drastically reduce the number of prenatal visits for Medicaid patients due to the funding cuts. As the 1996 welfare law changes are implemented, the number of poor families eligible for Medicaid is slowly but steadily dropping—currently at about one percent per month. Under the hostile state health care environment, Medicaid auditors have even refused to honor reimbursement rates that had earlier been promised in writing. The feeling among staff and board members is, "We are survivors. We will go on because we must."

Like many other Community Health Centers, Over 60 has survived because it fills a major community need that is not filled by other organizations. The clinic has gradually reinvented itself during its twenty-year history; it is not any single process or group of people that keeps it going. It was begun by a coalition of public spirited middle-class white and working-class black women, whose dedication and energy inspired others—students, young people of various races and classes, local officials—to help.

As time went by, the clinic had to grow and diversify in order to survive, and it needed an ever-increasing supply of professional expertise to do so. Talented nurses, physicians, community health workers, and administrators were attracted to the organization by the strength of its idealism, and the obvious need for its services in the community. In the process, the survival strategy evolved. It started with heavy reliance on small, informal, and local resources: cash donations, volunteer labor, neighborhood good will, patronage of city and county agencies and officials. It evolved toward reliance on much larger, more bureaucratic and remote resources: federal and state reimbursement programs and grants, regional and national foundations, contracts and alliances with large health care organizations and insurance companies.

In the process, it sometimes appears as though the word *community* as in *community health center* has ceased to apply to Over

60. Although a majority of the board are still users, very few users now understand more than a small fraction of the policies, procedures, or strategies that make the clinic run, or grasp the complex and changing economic and political forces to which it must respond month in and month out in order to survive. Richard Couto noticed a similar process in his study of small rural clinics in Tennessee and Kentucky in the 1970s:

> The health councils [that is, boards made up of local townspeople] are much more likely to be the stable element in the provision of health services, as administrators and staff members come and go. Yet we do far too little to stabilize the councils, train their members, and orient professionals to their authority in underserved areas. Instead, we make efforts to fit these councils and other community efforts into a health care system whose indifference and inherent defects necessitated community efforts in the first place. (1982, 99)

But it would be a mistake to think that the participation of the community has ceased to be important at Over 60. The users on the board continue to be quite aware of the needs, lifestyles, and attitudes of the clinic's clients, and make an effort to see that the administration and staff of the clinic, and its policies and plans, remain sensitive to those needs. Perhaps unlike some of the rural villages studied by Couto, there is an abundance of professional and administrative talent in a major city like Berkeley, from which an organization can draw staff whose ideals to some extent match their own.

Of even greater importance is the element of political and financial support for the clinic in the wider city and region. I believe that virtually everyone whose work has some potential impact on the clinic, from elected officials to hospital administrators to news editors to potential corporate donors, perceive Over 60 as one of the region's most popular institutions—both in the sense that it is widely admired, and in the sense that it is a true expression of the collective will of the community.

I think this perception is actually fairly accurate. The citizens of Alameda County probably know very little about the real health needs of the low-income elderly in their midst, or about how Over 60 goes about meeting those needs; but many of them know the clinic by reputation. They see favorable stories about it in the papers, they hear its name spoken approvingly by officials, they may know someone who has volunteered there, or made a donation. When they see a threadbare elderly person in the street they may think comfortingly to themselves, "We have a good clinic here for people like her."

And Over 60 continues to strive to deserve this reputation, by focusing its energies on a goal that, while it appears almost embarrassingly obvious, is at best an afterthought in the wider American health care system: to assure that its services are (a) appropriate for its clientele, and (b) accessible to everyone who needs them. This involves continuous, diligent efforts to assess client needs, to design services to meet those needs, and to secure funding to develop and sustain those services. The result of these efforts is an unusually well-coordinated, unusually broad array of carefully designed medical, environmental, and social services, many of which are not reimbursed by public or private health insurances.

In the fall of 1994 I interviewed two social workers and two physicians at Over 60, in an effort to learn more about the clinic's philosophy and style of working. The following stories about patients are condensed from those interviews.

Patricia

Patricia was described by the social worker as a character. She didn't trust doctors or any other institutional intrusions into her privacy. She would never have voluntarily come to Over 60, but the staff heard about her through a male friend who was worried about her. Like Patricia herself, the friend was clearly someone who cherished his independence, judging by his tattoos and other motorcyclist cultural markings. Patricia, he told the staff, was overweight, had very bad teeth, and didn't eat well. Also, she was dirt poor.

A visit from a social worker was unsuccessful; Patricia simply yelled at her through the closed door, telling her to go away. The biker friend agreed to help Patricia get food, and the social worker certified him for food stamps to this end.

The Over 60 staff persisted in trying to meet with Patricia, and with the help of the friend finally succeeded. She was of Italian descent, and had spent her life caring for other family members. She was now sixty-four, and everyone else in the family was dead. Patricia lacked the usual graces of someone used to society; her speech, for example, was of the type usually used by working-class males only among themselves.

Staff learned that she owned her own home and rented part of it out. Her neighborhood was plagued by robbery, and she had been victimized several times. Her relationship with her tenants was mutually hostile. Her distressed economic situation resulted in part from their frequent failure to pay the rent or utility bills.

Once a trusting relationship had been established between Patricia and the social worker, she allowed herself to be brought to the clinic for an assessment. Among many other problems, she was found to have uncontrolled diabetes. She was enrolled in Medicaid, but with impaired mobility and little money, she could not make regular trips to the clinic for treatment, so the staff arranged for home visits. The clinic delivered medications and supplies to her home, where she also received podiatric care. She was able to come to the clinic occasionally for dental treatment.

The social worker continued to work on Patricia's financial problems, with considerable success. She arranged for a local charity, Christmas in April, to repair and upgrade her home, and helped her find new tenants. At the time of the interview, both her health and her finances had stabilized.

Ralph

Ralph was the victim of a seizure disorder. He was unusually small and physically weak, and he had difficulty sustaining complex ideas. He walked with an impaired gait that reminded people of Charlie Chaplin. When he first came to the clinic he was only forty-nine, but he seemed to be a natural client for Over 60, since his problems required a comprehensive case management approach.

Ralph had a history of gambling, alcoholism, and suicide attempts. Because of his physical and cognitive limitations, he was on SSI and Medicaid, but he would go to the gambling casinos in Emeryville when his check came every month and lose much of his meager income. His only stable resource was a friend named Joe who had an apartment and allowed Ralph to sleep on his couch and scrounge from his refrigerator for two hundred dollars per month.

Ralph's situation worsened dramatically, then, when Joe had a stroke and was put in a nursing home. By the time he was discharged, Joe had decided to move to another apartment without Ralph. Lacking survival skills, Ralph was in danger of becoming homeless. After a good deal of searching, however, his social worker at Over 60 found him another apartment. This one was in a large building, and the social worker talked to the manager and to other residents about Ralph's problems. They agreed to look out for him. Some of the residents donated furniture for his apartment. He is able to get his meals in the common dining room, and one of the women residents does a bit of housekeeping for him on contract.

When I interviewed his social worker, Ralph had joined an adult day-care program that picked him up two days a week. With the support not only of the clinic and day-care center staff, but also his apartment neighbors, he has developed a new self-confidence. "He even has his own bank account now," said the social worker, "and since his apartment is a long way from Emeryville and he's so busy, he rarely goes to the casinos anymore."

Mrs. Brundage

In these cases the integrated social-medical approach might have made the difference not only between independence and institutionalization, but between life and death. But the approach sometimes has subtler applications. Some months after I collected the stories of Patricia and Ralph, I accompanied Over 60 nurse practitioner Natalia on a home visit to a ninety-nine-year-old black woman in west Berkeley.

The post-Victorian wood-frame house is somewhat larger than others in this predominantly African American neighborhood people call The Flats, but it does not stand out otherwise. Natalia takes a last minute look at Mrs. Brundage's chart, then picks up her medical bag, and we climb out of the car and head for the steps to the front door. The bell is answered by a man of wiry physique and receding hairline, dressed in jeans and a work shirt. "Hi," says Natalia, "I'm the nurse from Over 60, to see Mrs. Brundage?"

The inside of the house is a total surprise. Everything looks 1930s—furniture, wallpaper, pictures on the walls—all of it in perfect condition, as though it had not been touched in sixty years. Even the natural wood finish of the doors and baseboards looks new. I feel odd, almost like an intruder from another era. The man explains that he is Mrs. Brundage's nephew. As he escorts us through the museum-like interior to her room, he is quiet and a bit ill at ease, with the air of a person who doesn't really belong here either. Having delivered us at her bedroom door, he quickly excuses himself and disappears.

Mrs. Brundage is tiny, but aside from her white hair and stooped posture, she looks closer to sixty than to her real age— the skin of her face soft and smooth. She is dressed in an immaculate plain cotton shift, and a white sweater. She sits, regarding us curiously, on the edge of a bed that matches the antique decor. "Get a chair from the other room," she says to me. Meanwhile, Natalia, indicating a large carved chest near the bed, asks if she can sit there. "If you don't wiggle," says Mrs. Brundage. The room is comfortable and feminine, with flounces and big pillows. A matching pair of silhouettes hangs from long cords hooked to the ogee molding near the ceiling, but otherwise there is just the heavy furniture—a Spartan absence of the bric-a-brac and mementos that tend to fill long-occupied rooms. I notice that there is a blackened electrical outlet in the corner, as though some appliance had died dramatically here.

Natalia has not been here before. There is a moment of awkwardness as the interview begins; but Mrs. Brundage handles it like someone accustomed to such things. How is she getting on? "Oh, not so bad. I'm too crazy to go crazy," she says. Does she have difficulty with personal care? "I get dizzy when I go to make the bed." Does anyone help her with her chores? "When you can't do for yourself, your blood is poison to you," she says. Natalia asks whether, by "blood," she means family. Mrs. Brundage nods, and adds that she was living with a sister until two months ago, but that she "doesn't like that woman's ways." Her nephew shops for her, and she cooks for herself, except for lunch, which is delivered by meals-on-wheels.

The physical exam reveals that her systolic pressure is much too high (293), and that her feet and ankles are swollen and discolored. She keeps a shoebox of pills near her bed, among which are diuretics and blood pressure medications. She is supposed to take a "water pill" every other day, but she doesn't do it. Natalia gently brings the conversation back to this point several times, finally eliciting that Mrs. B doesn't like to take them, because she has difficulty getting to the toilet on time when she does.

The blood pressure, the swollen, purple feet, the noncompliance, the blackened electrical outlet. I begin to feel acutely uncomfortable about her situation: "This person could die!" But Natalia is serene. Will Mrs. Brundage take the pills if they are broken in half for her? She grudgingly agrees, and Natalia breaks them, then sticks a label on the bottle and writes in large letters: "1/2 TABLET EVERY OTHER DAY." "I'll see you next month," she says when the interview is finally over. We have been here forty-five minutes.

Following the exam, we say good-bye to Mrs. B sitting just as we found her on her bed, and go to look for the nephew. In his subdued manner, he tells us that she won't eat his cooking, and that he knows he is "not the favorite family member." The gas stove is no surprise: ancient but immaculate. A look in the refrigerator reveals leftover fried chicken and collard greens, and very little else.

Walking back to the car, I can't help offering suggestions. Maybe we could get a Friendly Caller to phone her regularly and remind her to take the medicine? Maybe someone could come and make suggestions about how to improve the safety of the house? Or talk to her about nutrition—it looks like she lives on salt and fat. Natalia smiles and says, "I don't know if Mrs. Brundage would respond well to suggestions from outsiders. Look at her. She's independent, she has her dignity, she's ninety-nine years old. She must be doing something right."

Troubled, I reflect on Natalia's words as we head back to the clinic along rainy streets. Perhaps discomfort, disability, and approaching death are integral parts of serene and dignified though fragile lives, carefully woven over many long years. Subtle differences in the quality and meaning of events can validate or mock those lives, making the difference between triumph and tragedy. To recognize the strength and intelligence with which Mrs. Brundage manages (I almost said "rules") her milieu, and to respect her choices, may be a far greater gift than the extra months of anxious life offered by the medical dragon-slayer. Of course, for someone else, the extra years of life—at whatever cost to one's dignity—might be the obvious choice.

To me, such stories illustrate what the word *community* in the phrase *community health center* means. By striving to know the values and lifestyles of its clients and the problems that interfere with their realization, the CHCs are more likely than other health organizations to provide that particular combination of services that make the most sense for a particular community. In the next chapter, we consider the social process that makes this possible.

Exercises and Study Questions

1. Why does the U.S. government play a smaller role in managing access to health care than most governments in the developed world? (This can be discussed in the form of a debate between public sector and private sector advocates.)

2. Suppose you are the director of a CHC in a middle-sized city. Your main clients are (a) homeless, (b) mothers and children on welfare, (c) uninsured workers, and (d) undocumented immigrants. How, and to whom, would you make your case for public support?

3. How are current economic trends (see especially chapters 4 and 5) likely to affect health care accessibility in future decades?

4. What have been the main arguments against public support of CHCs?

5. Talk to someone who is familiar with the health care system in one of the other industrial countries (Canada, the United Kingdom, Denmark, Japan). What are its strengths and weaknesses? Does it include ideas that might be tried in the United States?

Facilitating Community Involvement

CHAPTER 8

We have seen that the meaning of the word *community* tends to change as CHCs grow, consolidate their gains, and adapt to the wider political and economic environment. But to the extent that the community health center movement has succeeded in improving health care access for poor and underserved communities, it has done so by involving those communities themselves in the change process. People who live in the communities where the centers are located have to provide the knowledge of local issues and concerns that the clinics need. Local people also have to provide the leadership, the clientele, some of the capital, and most of the volunteer support base that is absolutely necessary at the outset.

In short, the health centers often have to participate in a process that includes some or all of these steps: (a) identifying a set of needs that are widely felt in the communities, (b) mobilizing energy needed to address those needs; (c) dealing with the inertia, fear, isolation, and cynicism that has prevented people from addressing those needs previously; (d) setting in motion a process that will get people with diverse ideas, backgrounds, and goals (and sometimes with long-standing antagonisms) to work together; (e) identifying the resources (material, talent, labor) available, both inside and outside the community, to support the development process; (f) dealing with the opposition to change that is sure to develop among those who gain the most from the status quo.

This process is necessarily unique in each community, since the needs, resources, obstacles, and personalities are different. There can be no blueprint for mobilizing a community to improve its health care system; but this does not mean that nothing has been learned that can be used to ease and speed the process of future efforts to serve the poor. In this chapter I will draw on what I and others have distilled from studying the process in a wide variety of settings.

What is a Community?

We have discussed some of the differences between traditional communities, where mutual knowledge among people is deep and interaction highly structured, and neighborhoods or towns in industrial societies, where anonymity is more the rule. Often in our society, one finds groups of people living in close proximity, who spontaneously band together to work cooperatively for a common cause, and it is usually this kind of group that we envision when we use the word *community*.

However, the word is often used by social planners and would-be leaders in a very different sense. It is used to refer to the potential that a group of neighbors is thought to have for carrying out some cooperative project that the planners and activists believe to be in the group's interest. Ordinarily, the concept of community-based health care makes sense because it seeks to make use of the fact that people whose lives and identities are interrelated (not necessarily peacefully) will, under the right conditions, participate to some extent collectively in decisions and in work; and this collectiveness can greatly increase the efficiency and effectiveness of health promotion efforts. The example we just presented of the Over 60 Health Center is a case in point.

It is this sense of the concept community that we generally find in the growing literature on community-based health care. In this literature one often sees such phrases as, "Planning must always involve community consultation," and "Nothing will succeed unless the community supports it" (see, for example, Brown 1997, 383). At first glance such statements seem sound, but as soon as we begin to think concretely about putting them into practice, we come up against problems.

First of all, it is clearly insufficient, for purposes of social change, to use the word for something as simple and tangible as a geographic area. There are many ways of defining a locality. There are villages, towns, city council districts, school districts, church parishes, urban boroughs and wards, and a host of informal designations referring to the areas around parks, commercial centers, social-class divisions, and so on. Locals may know more-or-less what the boundaries of The South Bronx, The Tenderloin, Little Havana, or Olivera Street are, but these boundaries usually split apart some groups of people who consider themselves neighbors or allies, and lump together others who have few common interests or relationships. Where should the lines of a given functional community be drawn? If we are searching for a cooperative reality, are the people we are searching for really related by geography at all, or is it ethnicity, social class, or religious or political affiliation that suggests their common interest?

This interrelatedness can be actual, in the sense that people regularly interact for some purpose or other, or it can be potential, in the sense that people would interact if they saw a good reason to do so. Consider a neighborhood where people living next door often speak to each other and to shopkeepers in their street, making friendly conversation or exchanging information about everyday concerns. They may rarely interact with, and not recognize, people from the next street over. But if some unusual event arises that affects the wider neighborhood—a disaster, or a threat to people's well-being, for example—they will work together because they are capable of thinking of themselves collectively as a neighborhood for this limited purpose. In the process of working together, they discover things about each other that make it easier to communicate: common cultural or geographic origins, tastes, beliefs, interests, and so on, and the boundaries of the neighborhood may shift as a result.

A different scenario might involve a small rural community or suburb. Here, people know a fair amount about each other, and may be accustomed to socializing at church, school, and so on. They may think of themselves as belonging to certain well-defined subgroups within the town, such as parents of young children, members of an ethnic group or church, or the country club set. Cooperation is more likely to follow these lines of self-identification than lines of individual motivation.

However, in both settings, some individuals will have a stronger interest in a given problem or issue. If the issue involves public safety or education, for example, parents will generally come forward. Also, some people are simply more community minded than others, or have more time to work on collective projects. Individuals will get involved for a great variety of reasons—political ambition, altruism, loneliness, curiosity, commercial interests, family sentiments, ethnic or class loyalty, vindictiveness, friendship, romantic attraction, or simple boredom. People's beliefs about the specific problem at hand, and about the process of its solution, will have a major effect on whether and how they become involved as well—whether, for example, they believe improvement is both possible and important, given the situation; whether they identify with the leadership; and who they think will benefit most from a particular solution.

Also in both settings residents are likely to discover during the communicative process (if they did not already know) that there are several subgroups of people among them who have very different ideas about what ought to be done, and these subgroups will form competing divisions that make cooperative work more difficult. Meanwhile, those active within the community will discover that there are others outside it who may either help or hinder the cooperative work; and linkages to these outsiders become part of the community process.

In short, where there is no ready-made cooperative process in place, the potential for community work will affect different individuals, families, and institutions both within and beyond the local geographic area differently. People will act partly on the basis of knowledge and belief, partly on the basis of interest, and partly on the basis of self-identification. It might be very hard to predict by geography, by social class, or by any other characteristic, who will get involved in a given issue or in what way—who, in other words, the community will actually turn out to be. The questions of what will emerge as the interests and goals of that community, what competing views will emerge, or which of those views will prove more powerful, are even less predictable.

An effective approach to community involvement in the absence of a well-organized effort, then, requires knowledge about two kinds of things: first, exactly how the concept of community cooperation is relevant to the activist's work; and second, how to describe the process (in terms of actors, actions, institutions, and issues) that will bring that relevance to life. One useful way of thinking about the meaning of community is to reframe the concept, from one of locale to one of process. In other words, the health care activist is searching, not so much for a community of people, as for a process of community formation and cooperation. As Cheryl Walter (1997) says, community for the change agent is a "milieu," not a "place."

What does it mean, then, to say that successful community change must begin "where the people are," or must take the "community's needs and values" into account? The answer to this question, again, while extremely important from both an ethical and a practical point of view, turns out to be far from simple. These notions refer to an emergent process, in which the community in question comes into being, to some extent, in response to a vision of change; but at the same time, that vision must be shaped by the needs, values, and perceptions of the people who will bring it into being. As a process that evolves out of itself, each example of it is in some ways unique and it cannot be adequately described once and for all. Stewardship of community-based social change must always be open to redefinition of goals and methods. However, we can try to conceptualize the process a bit more concretely:

1. Preliminary definition by change agent(s) of a desired state of affairs either for a defined population or a defined locale, that might be achieved by cooperation among some residents and institutions in that locale. This definition should seek to specify to some extent, who (social characteristics) stands to gain or lose what (objective values), if this state of affairs should be effected. In other words, what are the stakes and who are the stakeholders.

2. Collection of preliminary information about the shared needs, beliefs, feelings, and resources relevant to the vision of every definable group of stakeholders.

3. Negotiation among the change agent(s) and stakeholders concerning who will participate, in what way, and toward what jointly supported goals. (Note: This step is absolutely crucial. A common mistake in organizing is to listen to the most vocal or accessible people in the community, and overlook those whose views and participation are hard to elicit, but nonetheless essential for success.)

4. Formation of a process whereby the commitments of all participants to the goals and to the process can be monitored and the results fed back into the direction and methods of the project.

The Role of the Health Professional I: Competence and Responsibility

There are two major ethical dilemmas that face the health professional as a social change agent. One is to reconcile professional competence with social responsibility. The other is to reconcile professional power with client autonomy. Let us discuss these in turn.

In chapter 1 I touched on the problem of whether health work—and therefore professionalism in the health sciences—should include awareness of the social causes of ill health, and leadership in addressing those causes. I mentioned that this is a subject of passionate debate in medicine and, to a lesser extent, in nursing and other health professions. A casual survey of articles and editorials in the leading health science journals reveals a full spectrum of opinion from within the professions—from a strictly private and individualistic approach to a vigorous social activist one.

At the individualistic end of the continuum, one finds the following kinds of statements:

> Both established patients of a [community-oriented primary care] practice and the total community have an interest that the physician provide personal care. *Providing such care is*

the societal role of the physician, and society gives the physician special rewards and dispensations for being in that role. If that role is abandoned, no one else will fill it for the physician's patients.

On the other hand, the total community . . . would potentially benefit by a [community-oriented primary care] program. (Freeman 1987, 377; emphasis added)

Freeman concludes that the physician is justified in devoting time to collective community health concerns, as long as service to no individual patient is directly compromised by such work.

A somewhat more activist position is that health professionals have both special knowledge about the health effects of certain political policies or social attitudes, and collective political power by virtue of their widely accepted advisory role. Accordingly, they have an opportunity to educate policy makers and the public about serious health-related political issues. This is the position taken with respect to nuclear weapons, for example, by Arnold Relman, editor of the *New England Journal of Medicine*: "I have suggested before that in pressing for this goal [of nuclear stockpile reduction], physicians will be most effective if they remain largely united. Such consensus is not likely to be maintained unless we concentrate on our educational role and advocate broad policies that follow from the medical and scientific considerations and can win support of rational people in all political camps" (Relman 1986, 890).

A still more activist position says that health professionals not only have an opportunity to make social changes, they have an obligation to do so—first, by increasing their knowledge of social problems, then by advocating for their solutions. Weinreb and Bassuk, for example, conclude that practitioners and teachers of family medicine should play a leadership role in studying the needs of homeless families and in developing curricula for the training of other professionals in dealing with those needs, and should join other professionals in advocating for public policies to address those needs.

Family medicine's long tradition of working with underserved patients, its clinical expertise . . . and its knowledge of family assessment and functioning place it in a unique position to assume a leadership role in working with homeless families. Through direct service, medical education, clinical research, and advocacy, family medicine can help many families and contribute significantly to eradicating homelessness. (Weinreb and Bassuk 1990, 79)

Finally, a few professional commentators encourage us to see the health provider not simply as a knowledgeable outsider, advocating on behalf of the dispossessed, but as their trusted ally whose mission of healing is best served "by putting their skills at the disposal of those acting with the poorest and most powerless . . . encouraging democratic control over the provision of health care and showing oneself willing to submit to the will of the majority, rather than asserting one's professional autonomy" (Sanders and Carver 1985, 219).

All of these points of view allow some attention to social causes as an integral function of the health professional, and I offer them as a sampling from which to draw in choosing one's own identity and role. What is effective and personally satisfying for one health worker might be awkward and personally difficult for another, depending on one's character and skills, and the social reality in which one finds oneself.

My experience working in community health, however, indicates that health care professionals, by virtue of their knowledge and the confidence placed in them by others, often can contribute to the search for community-based solutions to health problems in a wide variety of ways. Some of these ways may expose the health worker to serious criticism from those with other ways of thinking. Some, however, appear to me to fall well within the limits of ordinary citizen participation in community life.

Of course, the degree and kind of appropriate social action that a health worker takes will depend on his or her knowledge of (a) the community in question (see chapter 3) and communities like it; (b) the types of clientele and health problems in question; (c) the institutions (clinic, hospital, school, nursing home, church, local government, charitable organization, and so on) involved; (d) the individuals (clients, civic leaders, health care managers) involved; (e) the dynamics of social change in settings of this type.

Without trying to give an exhaustive list of possible roles, then, here are some that come to mind:

- Identify and network individually with leaders in the community—health professionals, public officials, journalists, teachers, business leaders—who are interested in social approaches to improving health.

- Actively volunteer (as board member, advisor, research assistant, health provider) in an ongoing organization (consumer group, community clinic, health commission, self-help group) interested in such approaches.

- Seek paid employment in a setting that aims at socially conscious health solutions, such as community clinics and client-centered organizations (unions, nonprofit community groups, church-based projects, and so forth).

- Serve as an advocate (write letters and make phone calls, testify at hearings, lobby public officials) for client groups on local, state, and national issues affecting health (housing, sanitation, jobs, education, transportation, pay and working conditions, health insurance).

- Take a leadership role in stimulating community involvement in health care.

The Role of the Health Professional II: Power and Autonomy

In chapter 1 I also discussed the problem of the power gap that usually separates health providers from poor clients. This gap becomes even more problematic when the health professional assumes a position of leadership in a community. Often, the professional not only wields the symbols of superior knowledge of health and illness, and the power to access needed health care institutions and technologies. He or she is also likely to hold some keys to financial and political power that can have major effects on the lives of communities.

Assuming that the socially responsible health worker shares the egalitarian values of most social activists, these power differentials set up a number of ethical traps that bear careful thought.

- Community members may defer to the health worker out of lack of self-confidence, or politeness, rather than conviction. The impact of the project might then be a lowering of local self-esteem and efficacy.
- Some community members might take pride in refusing to be influenced by a powerful outsider. The self-esteem of some might thrive at the expense of real solutions for others.
- The health worker might be competing unwittingly with promising people and issues, thereby replacing local capacity with external help.

  Or some locals might be led to cultivate a relationship with the health worker or the project in order to improve their own position or further their own agenda. The result might be the loss of effectiveness and self-esteem by the losers in community power struggles.
- Other outsiders might seek to use the health worker's presence to legitimate their own ends, either as professed allies of the project or as its antagonists.

All of these possibilities (and there are doubtless others) underline the moral responsibility of the health worker to be maximally conscious, not only of one's own power, but of the role of power in general within the community. Much more might be at stake than the success or failure of the project itself. Some specific questions that need to be studied in any effort at social change are the following:

- What are the main viewpoints on critical social issues in the community? Who holds them? What are the affiliations (both internal and external) and resources of each key group or player?
- How is power and prestige negotiated in the community? What leads to political success or failure, and why?
- Who holds the bulk of the power and resources needed to either promote or hinder the project? What are the stakes for each person or group?
- What is the history of relations among the various potential stakeholders? How is this history likely to affect their future relations?

- What is the history of relations between the community and outsiders with similar agendas? What worked, what didn't work, and why?

Having a sense of these issues will not guarantee that intervention will produce beneficial results, or even avoid harmful ones. But such knowledge can help the community health activist assess the wisdom of intervening in the power dynamics of a community in a particular way. Sometimes, one has to take risks, but the decision to do so should be as morally conscious as possible.

Community Involvement: Awareness

When I first began working with community groups (in Honduras in 1993), I expected people to be eager to cooperate for better health. It is not difficult to understand that improvements in neighborhood sanitation and water supply, and access to immunization, basic medicines, and screening, is likely to help everyone. All that would be needed, I thought, would be some information about what the community's most serious health problems were, and some assistance in organizing to address these.

To my dismay, I found that most people, most of the time, are not very interested in community health—or not interested enough to divert serious energy into improving it. In Honduras as in other places where I have worked, people understood immediately that neighborhood child nutrition could be improved by bulk purchasing of powdered milk, that worms and infections could be reduced by digging latrines, or that lobbying local officials for a communal deep well could save both lives and money. Getting them to unite to do these things was the difficult thing.

Part of the problem is that most people who are likely to take action on any such issue are (a) not sick most of the time, and (b) busy doing other things. Without a secure food supply, hunger cannot be ignored; without secure shelter, housing becomes a priority; if one lives in constant fear of violence, safety is a must. These problems are so pressing that a community cannot ignore them if they are widespread. However, except during epidemics, ill health is an occasional personal problem, and one that individuals may not notice much when it affects their neighbors. As every nurse or physician knows, even those who have chronic or recurring health problems get used to them over time. Often victims have to be persuaded to seek treatment.

The first challenge of community involvement in health, often, is to raise awareness of the problems. If we look at how this has been done successfully, we see two related principles. (1) Start where awareness is, then let connections to health follow. (2) Create opportunities to reinforce awareness of health.

Start Where Awareness Is

Observing a poor community, and even talking casually with people in it, one often gets the impression that there is very little awareness of shared problems. People feel personally oppressed, but also feel powerless to do anything about it, or even afraid to discuss it, except with family. A public health worker studying environmental problems in the slums of Glasgow told me that in addition to deplorable housing and unemployment, there were serious sanitation problems, poor schools, and a lack of transportation in some neighborhoods. But those were not what got public attention. Rather, everyone wanted to talk about dog poop: the fact that too many people let their pets defecate in the street.

The poor often get the message from the wider society that they have no useful knowledge or opinions—that knowledge belongs to people who are educated, or who have positions and titles of respect. This message is likely to be especially strong when the poor want to challenge the accepted way of doing things. There are many organizations in this country—some national and some local—that work tirelessly to combat this situation, but these organizations (for example, the Urban League, the NAACP, Highlander Center, the local income and welfare rights organizations and social justice commissions) are for the most part shut out of the mainstream media, and knowledge about them is quite limited. As a result of all these factors, the shared problems of poor communities simply go unsolved, often for many years.

Several kinds of experiences can change this, sometimes liberating a surprising store of knowledge and energy. Often local awareness of injustices and problems is given voice and organization by national social movements, as was the case during the Civil Rights Movement in the rural South. When blacks in the South first heard Stokely Carmichael and Martin Luther King, many knew immediately that their own problems were being voiced by these leaders, and began to discuss the issues and their remedies with their neighbors. Given the climate of change, the result was often a dramatic, collective revisioning of the community and its needs (Couto 1991).

But usually there is no social movement on the horizon, and change must begin from within. A technique for beginning this change that has been used very effectively by unions, civil rights groups, and public health workers alike is simply to begin by creating a forum—a safe and accessible place—for people to come together to talk. A successful maternal health project in a low-income neighborhood in Richmond, California, began by responding to the needs young women expressed in group meetings, and creating a handicraft project where they could learn skills to generate extra income. Once they saw that they could (a) change things, and (b) trust the health workers, they were ready to take on health projects. This method is described in detail in the works of such social reformers as Highlander Folk School founder Myles Horton (Adams 1975) and adult educator Paulo Freire (1970).

In essence, when people learn from each other that their problems are not private but shared by the community, they overcome their shame and are able to discuss both the problems and the solutions more openly. Through the process of listening and being listened to sympathetically, they begin to build trust and sympathy not only for one another, but for themselves as well. Finally, through thinking and acting collectively, they lose much of the fear that attended the idea of acting alone. Being able to take courageous action then raises the whole process to a new level of self-respect and hope.

Throughout this process, it is crucial that the facilitator should

- nurture burgeoning self-respect by validating participants' experience and ideas, and by taking a nondirective role;
- nurture equality and harmony within the community by

avoiding favoritism, and by encouraging mutual respect on all sides;

- foster trust among participants—and between them and one-self—by modeling and encouraging openness, honesty, and good faith.

In his book on the subject, Ernest Stringer lists the Working Principles of Community-Based Action Research—a list that applies perfectly to the role of the change facilitator. Stringer divides his principles into four areas: relationships, communication, participation, and inclusion, as follows:

Relationships in action research should
- Promote feelings of *equality* for all people involved
- Maintain *harmony*
- *Avoid conflicts* where possible
- *Resolve conflicts* that arise, openly and dialogically
- *Accept* people as they are, not as some people think they ought to be
- Encourage *personal, cooperative relationships*, rather than impersonal, competitive, conflictual, or authoritarian relationships
- Be *sensitive* to people's feelings

In effective *communication*, one
- Listens *attentively* to people
- *Accepts* and trusts what they say
- Can be *understood* by everyone
- Is *truthful and sincere*
- Acts in socially and *culturally appropriate ways*
- Regularly *advises* others about what is happening

Participation is most effective when it
- Enables significant levels of active *involvement*
- Enables people to *perform* significant tasks
- Provides *support* for people as they learn to act for themselves
- Encourages plans and activities that people are able to *accomplish* themselves
- Deals *personally* with people rather than with their representatives or agents

Inclusion in action research involves

- Maximization of the involvement of *all* relevant *individuals*
- Inclusion of *all groups* affected
- Inclusion of *all relevant issues*—social, economic, cultural, political—rather than a focus on narrower administrative or political agendas
- Ensuring *cooperation* with other groups, agencies, and organizations
- Ensuring that all relevant groups *benefit* from activities (Stringer 1996, 38)

These things can be difficult to do. The community or its individual participants might

- begin by focusing on problems the facilitator thinks are irrelevant
- embark on plans that appear self-defeating
- take a long time to make seemingly simple decisions, or bog down in petty disagreements
- exert strong pressure on the facilitator to take a directive role
- grant leadership to people with whom the facilitator disagrees
- fail to follow through on plans or live up to commitments, thereby undermining the facilitator's trust
- periodically lose self-confidence and momentum, or need extra encouragement

Unfortunately, in my experience, there is no magic solution to these problems. There does not seem to be an effective alternative to the empowerment process for generating significant and lasting social change; and improving community health may depend on such change. For this reason, being a successful facilitator of community change generally requires a major commitment of energy over a long period (at least months, more often years).

It also requires genuine humility. As I said, health is not often one of the uppermost social/economic issues for the majority of people in poor communities; and the health professional must often suspend his or her sense of professional authority and become "one of the worker bees," showing good faith and supporting the growth of autonomy by accepting (within the limits of one's conscience) nonprofessional leadership, ideas, and goals. The rewards of success, of course, might be enormous.

Create Opportunities for Awareness of Health

The principles of local autonomy, equality, and inclusiveness are necessary in directed social change because they are the principles that foster a sense of mutual caring—of citizenship—in a community. When people feel listened to, respected, and supported regardless of their social position, they begin to reciprocate. If the process is strong enough and long enough, the most active people in the community will be those who adhere most strongly to these values.

Once this happens, health will eventually emerge as a focus of awareness among the activists. For one thing, the attitude of citizenship (meaning mutual caring, not jingoism) invariably promotes concern for the weakest and neediest—children, the frail elderly, the sick, the disabled, the poor, victims of injustice. Communal awareness is likely to begin with the problems that affect the largest number of people, such as crime, joblessness, political oppression, or pollution. But if health care is inadequate for the most vulnerable (and where isn't it!) it will become part of the agenda, even if it is not given top priority.

Moreover, at some time or other both curative and preventive health care affects everyone, either personally or through close relationships. Having needed care ourselves or having a loved one who does, we find the needs of the sick understandable. Most of us also know the fear of illness, and can recognize at least some of the health hazards around us.

I have said that the role of the activist health professional is not to set the agenda for the community. But one can help the community make decisions by raising consciousness of health problems. One way to do this is through health fairs—free mass screenings resulting in new information on the prevalence of health problems. Done properly so that rates of participation are high, participants are satisfied with the service, and local leadership is thoroughly involved and informed, health fairs can change public awareness dramatically (see Couto 1982).

Other ways to increase awareness are (1) to encourage community members who have special knowledge of health issues, such as those who have health problems themselves, or who care for an ill or disabled person, to be active in leadership; (2) to educate the leadership oneself, using published statistics on local health (for a list of techniques and sources, see Nutting 1990, 161–242); (3) to encourage contact (through formal or informal meetings, speaking invitations, educational tours) between local leaders and those of other communities that have successfully addressed health problems.

Community Involvement: Leadership

The health professional involved in facilitating social change might be entering a process that is already well under way, with a well-defined cast of characters, a set of goals, and a way of operating; or, she may be among those who initiate the change process and play a role in deciding how it will be organized, and by whom. In either case, it is probably useful to know something about how inclusive, egalitarian, participatory group leadership functions, and what some of its pitfalls are.

No matter how a voluntary group is organized, and however well it seems to get work done, it has to cope with difficult problems stemming from the relationships of the people in it—the people who make the decisions and do the work. Over the past fifteen years I have participated in several voluntary groups organized on the principles of equality and inclusiveness described above; and in some more hierarchically organized groups as well—ones where there was a clear leadership structure, and decisions were made by majority vote rather than by consensus. In all these groups, the combination of voluntariness and group solidarity produced an insoluble paradox. On the one hand, in order to remain committed to the group, each individual volunteer needed to feel that what was done collectively truly represented what he or she believed in. To put it another way, each person in the group had a personal vision of what the group should accomplish, and how. What sustained participants' commitment and drew forth their energy was their perception that the group was implementing their personal vision, at least part of the time. This meant that the group had to struggle constantly to understand each member's personal vision, and do its best to implement that vision without unduly compromising the visions of the others. If the group strayed too far from a member's ideals for too long, that member would drop out, or even take action against the group.

On the other hand, none of these groups could have functioned collectively, unless each member had been willing to make compromises in their personal vision for the sake of group solidarity. Although there was much overlap between personal visions (otherwise the groups never would have coalesced in the first place), they were not quite the same. In other words, the solidarity of the group itself had to be one of the personal goals of all the people in it. The alternative would be a constant battle for control that would paralyze the group or even lead to its dissolution.[1]

If the activist health worker enters a voluntary group that is already functioning, presumably the group has found its way to a workable strategy for managing this dilemma. It would be well for the newcomer to try to understand what that strategy is, and why it is successful. However, if the group is just being formed, its founders have to contemplate various strategies. Should the group be a completely egalitarian and totally inclusive democracy, where anyone can participate who wants to, and where all decisions are made by consensus? Or should it be a closed collective, which strictly limits participation to those with the skills and values that match a preset array of needs? Or should it be a parliamentary democracy, with elected officials, a formal decision-making procedure, and majority rule? As the participants in a group get to know each other, they tend to give up rigid codes of procedure and do whatever the immediate situation seems to call for, sometimes shifting easily from egalitarianism to hierarchy and back.

It should help any community activist to know some of the pros and cons of the various forms of democracy commonly found in voluntary organizations. Assuming that none of my readers would be tempted to join a dictatorship or an oligarchy, let me contrast, then, the radically egalitarian form of organization sometimes called the *consensus group* with the more centrally organized *formal democracy*. The comments that follow are drawn partly from my own experience, and partly from Jane Mansbridge's excellent essay on the subject (Mansbridge 1973).

A consensus group (which in Mansbridge is called a *participatory group*) in its most radical form is one in which there is no fixed formal leadership, but an expectation that all members will share leadership roles equally. The ideal membership includes anyone who wants to participate, and the ideal process is one in which no decision is taken until everyone in the group agrees to it. What I am calling a formal democracy is a group in which membership is limited by certain qualifications (for example, local residence, gender), specific functions are done by formally appointed officers and committees, and decisions are arrived at by majority vote if consensus is lacking.

First I want to emphasize that the distinction between group types is sometimes trivial in practice, because groups that have worked together for some time tend to abandon formality and vary procedures to fit the moment. Groups founded on consensus principles often have strong leaders who direct most of the work, and formal democracies often operate as though roles are interchangeable and votes are unnecessary. Still, the difference in styles can be crucial, as I will try to show.

Consensus groups have the great virtue, which I mentioned in my discussion of awareness building, that they stimulate self-confidence and mutual trust among people who need these things in order to find the motivation to act. A number of studies have also been done on the dynamics of consensus groups, with interesting results. They have been shown to be more innovative, to produce more creative results and more daring decisions, and to lead to more correct answers to complex problems than formal democracies. The consensus group format also increases people's commitment to a decision, and makes members more likely to take action—especially risky action—on group decisions. It increases participants' general sense of mastery, that is, their sense that their environment can be made to respond positively to their own actions (Mansbridge 1973, 352–353).

On the down side, consensus groups often take more time commitment from their active members than other democracies, they stimulate members to express more feelings—including negative feelings—and they often fail to distribute power and re-spect as evenly as they pretend. Each of these problems is inti-mately entangled with the others in practice, but Mansbridge discusses them, for didactic purposes, as separate issues.

Time

When everyone in a group provides input into identifying and solv-ing problems, some progress still can be made by individual mem-bers outside group meetings, but more time is spent discussing each detail of each decision within meetings. Work can only pro-ceed when all persons have contributed what they think they have to offer, and when each is satisfied that he or she understands what the others are saying. Ironing out differences in viewpoint can be quite time consuming as well.

- This may discourage members who have already thought through the situation thoroughly and must hear all their own steps repeated, questioned, and explained.
- Many people also value action itself over their own feelings or their co-members', and lose interest in the social-emotional process long before it is over.
- Some participants might simply be too busy to stay with the process week in and week out.

As they accumulate experience working together, however, partici-patory groups can greatly reduce time to decide, while retaining accuracy, commitment, and morale. If members spend enjoyable time together outside of meetings, getting to know more about one another and attending to one another in a social way, the efficiency of group work time also tends to improve.

Emotion

Because consensus groups make a point of valuing the feelings and personalities of their members, and not just their intellectual con-tributions, ideas become closely linked with people and emotions. The good thing about this is that it nourishes commitment of people to each other, and to the ideas and ideals of the group. It makes people feel valued and boosts self-esteem and confidence. But there are also problems with it:

- People in small consensus groups often choose emotionally satisfying decisions over efficient ones. They may adopt ideas or promote individuals in order to be supportive, for example, knowing that a different decision would advance the objective work of the group better.

- The personal characteristics of members, such as their personalities or their symbolic significance for the group, may decide which ideas get listened to, rather than the objective value of what the opinion-leaders say. This can cause resentment to build up in others, who feel they are being slighted, occasionally even threatening to split the group.

- People who are uncomfortable with emotional confrontation, or uninterested in the work of mediating and repairing feelings, can feel acutely uncomfortable in such settings, and lose enthusiasm for the group.

- The mediating and repairing process can be exhausting, even for those who are comfortable. Occasionally, groups become so absorbed in the business of managing feelings that their original goals can get pushed aside for weeks at a time.

- Because each member of the group is given equal respect regardless of their views, a member or subgroup that insists on promoting ideas that are viewed negatively by the majority can produce a crisis; either forcing the group to banish him/them, or causing the group itself to break up.

Using a facilitator to broker the emotional process can be helpful.

Inequality

Any group brings together people with different levels of skill, experience, social capital, energy, and personal charisma. This fact tends to lead to the formation of an informal status hierarchy, even in the most assiduously egalitarian of groups. Inequality also slows down group work, because those with fewer skills or less information must be brought along by the more gifted or informed ones.

- People who end up lower on the hierarchy, those with less influence, will lose commitment unless they are made to feel needed.

- More influential members may lose interest if they have to go over the same ground again and again.

- Among residents of low-income communities where resources are always in short supply, control over the human power, money, facilities, or public voice of a small organization confers high prestige. Any tendency to monopolize any of these things by a member or faction of the group is likely to generate serious resentment from other members in such a community.

If the group is to adhere to its ideals of mutual respect, some attention must be paid to leveling out inequalities. One remedy is to structure time for teaching the less-skilled, less-informed members. If they can be taught how to get, analyze, and present information, for example, their participation will become more central. Another method is to look for tasks that will match the skill of members. For example, a member of a health center planning group might have few administrative skills, but might be able to get entree into neighborhoods where the center needs to organize residents or recruit users and donors.

The organization of group meetings can also be used to generate involvement. Small breakout groups give each member more chance to speak. A rotating chairmanship gives each member a turn in the limelight. Finally, the issue of inequality itself can be faced directly by the group. For example, a discussion of the needs and expectations of members might result in a decision to accept equality of respect as a principle, and forego equality of influence.

The Best Times, the Worst Times: Phases, Dilemmas, and Heroism

Becoming conscious of its own needs and its own potentials is a highly rewarding process for a community. In place of isolation and helplessness, people begin to find comradeship and personal strength. The leaders' newfound energy is infectious, and even those on the periphery chip in with whatever money or work they can spare. In the beginning, people see only the positive possibilities of their ideas, having not yet tested their limitations. In this phase, impoverished communities in Tennessee and Virginia raised tens of thousands of dollars through bake sales and raffles to build their clinics, leading Couto to characterize this as "the best times" (Couto 1982, 54). The Over 60 CHC started in much the same way: a handful of elderly women lobbying local government for resources and permits, going door to door to encourage potential users and ask for small donations, and holding endless potlucks, raffles, and picnics to raise awareness and money.

Sooner or later, this process begins to affect the power dynamics in a community. When poor people find they can change things, there is a lot they want changed. They want not only a fair share of local resources, they want to be represented in managing those resources. They want not only equal protection under the law, they want to influence the making of that law. They want not only better health care, they want a voice in deciding what health care is. They enter the phase of struggle—what Couto called "the worst times."

Early in this phase, people discover that hard work, solidarity, and good intentions are not enough; that one needs considerable skill and courage to anticipate and deal with the opposition of other stakeholders. They learn that some people who encouraged them at first will turn against them once they see the results; that some whose help they counted on want control of the project; that some who are hostile will stop at nothing to get their way. As problems become more complex, the advice of outside experts becomes crucial, creating new problems. It might be difficult to find such professionals who are comfortable taking direction from housewives, farmers, or auto mechanics. Potential lenders may want to dictate board qualifications. Government agencies might require drastic policy changes in return for grants, threatening the energy-sustaining vision of the project's founders. The people whose energy, grassroots reputation, and grasp of local needs brought the project to its flowering might have to be succeeded in power by people who can deal with the sheer complexity of clinic management and finance.

During the worst times, a tension usually develops between

means and ends—between the necessity of thriving financially and the necessity of sustaining the mission, which is the source of community support. Should a clinic dedicated to free access begin to charge user fees to stay solvent? Should one dedicated to the local neighborhood merge with a citywide or countywide organization in order to stabilize its budget? Should a health center add services that are easily funded, and defer adding riskier ones more needed by its main clientele? Should the organization risk negative publicity by joining in a rowdy public demonstration for a sympathetic cause?

The dilemmas of community-based groups, dilemmas not faced by profit-driven organizations, dramatize their true character and value: They are links between the situated moral values of communities on one hand and the rationalist-universalist values of industrial capitalist society on the other hand. The communal group strives to achieve at least an equality of respect by appealing to man's natural capacity for empathy. At most it strives for an all-inclusive moral consensus, something that implies not only equal respect but equal voice as well. Respect implies understanding—not analytic understanding, which is critical in nature, but empathic understanding, which is uncritical.

But as I mentioned in my discussion of community, there are no autonomous localities. Perhaps there never were. The community-based group must face outward, must participate in the wider society. This wider society also calls for respect—respect of values that are held to be rational and universal (such as money). Personal respect and voice are allotted in this wider sphere according to analytic understanding—the understanding of talents, knowledge, and resources. This is not a soft respect that leads to consensus, but a hard one that leads to competition—a respect for Darwinian fitness.

The community-based group constitutes itself for the purpose of representing the soft values of community, not just to its constituents (who are members of the wider society too), but to the *homo economicus* and his institutions in the wider society. In doing so, it performs a heroic service in both directions, demonstrating to society and the individual the truth of compassionate respect. I call it heroic because, embracing the weak, it puts itself at a disadvantage in the rational pursuit of strength. It is the beauty of this heroism that powers participation in, and support of, community-based groups. The group that chooses rational-universal values at the expense of compassionate respect thereby forfeits a large share of its power.

I began this book by saying that poverty is a moral phenomenon, and that it results from the failure of community. We have now come full circle. I am saying that the health worker can best address the needs of poor clients by practicing in a way that seeks to restore community values. Community clinics, I believe, are generally good ways to do that, but they are certainly not the only way.

Exercises and Study Questions

1. If you have ever been in the leadership of an organization
   - What was the leadership style: consensus, or formal democracy?
   - What was the most difficult thing about participating?
   - What was the most rewarding thing?
   - What were the main strengths and weaknesses of the organization?
   - In your view, how could it have been run more effectively?

2. Identify a major health problem in the area where you live or work that might be addressed by community involvement.
   - How would you define the community who might address this problem?
   - How would you begin to facilitate the involvement of this community in working on the problem? What problems would you foresee, and how would you approach them?

3. One of the greatest difficulties in facilitating community change is the amount of time it requires. Get together with others who might be interested in being change facilitators, and talk about ways to make time available in your lives for this kind of work.

APPENDIX A

INTERNET RESOURCES FOR

THE STUDY OF POVERTY

The details of poverty in the United States change rather rapidly, and those given in this book will soon be outdated. In order to be effective as a planner of health services and as an advocate for the poor, one needs to stay abreast of the latest developments.

Moreover, every state and local area has its own resources—clinics, shelters, legal and financial aid centers, advocacy groups—that can help the health care activist address local problems.

Probably the best way to access information that is up-to-date and pertinent to one's local area is to search the internet. If you do not have internet access yourself, you might be able to get it with the help of your local library, university, or health care facility. There is so much information on the internet, and it changes so rapidly, that here I can only point to a few sites that might help students get started, and develop their own list of favorite sites.

Asian Pacific Islander American Health Forum

www.igc.org/apiahf/pover.html APIA/HF is an advocacy organization for the health of Asian and Pacific Islander communities in America, but its site is broadly useful for health rights activists. It gives census data on poverty and health insurance, for example, and also has links to other information sites.

The Body

www.thebody.com An excellent resource for information on AIDS. This site has links to resources for getting help, to information about prevention and treatment, and to health care rights. You can even search for lists of AIDS help organizations in your city.

Bureau of Primary Health Care, U.S. Public Health Service

www.bphc.hrsa.dhhs.gov The Bureau is the main federal agency that supports the work of community clinics. Its excellent web site links to PHC organizations all over the country, as well as statistics and bibliography on community clinics.

California Primary Care Association

www.cpca.org This site has links to state and federal agencies of all kinds having information on primary health and health care. It is a good place to get information on community clinics and health rights legislation issues.

Health Care Financing Administration

www.hcfa.gov Provides information about Medicaid and Medicare, including eligibility criteria and services provided. This site also has a question-and-answer format, whereby you can get information on specific problems, such as how to appeal a claims denial.

Healthy Cities Project

www.healthycities.org Among other things, the Healthy Cities Project helps community groups work on health access issues, and produces policy documents on health equity. This site also has links to many organizations, and to specific Healthy Cities projects in many parts of the world.

Kaiser Family Foundation

www.kff.org This is a super site. It contains links to dozens of government and private organizations, university programs, and foundations at the national and state levels dealing with statistics on health, health rights issues and legislation, and new findings on the health of the poor. It also lists Kaiser Family Foundation projects of interest, and contains an extensive library catalogue, searchable by topic and document type.

Medicare, State by State

www.medicare.gov This U.S. Government site has links to all state Medicare offices, where you can find detailed information on Medicare rules and procedures in your locality.

National Association of Community Health Centers (NACHC)

www.nachc.com You have to be a member of NACHC to get past the home page. If you do not want to join, perhaps you can get access through your local community clinic. There is a great deal of information here on the work of community clinics and the people they serve.

National Coalition for the Homeless

http://nch.ari.net This is a nongovernmental organization that advocates for the homeless. Its site lists local and national private and government organizations and programs for the homeless. One can also get access to documents and statistics on homelessness here.

National Mental Health Association

www.nmha.org A mental health consumer rights organization, NMHA lists detailed information on mental health service users' rights, and lists help and information sources.

U.S. Census Search

www.census.gov/search97cgi/97_cgi The Census Bureau site lists resources on poverty and health census data. If you have Adobe Acrobat program, you can download documents.

Browse

I find that I get hundreds of interesting web results with descriptors like "Poverty and Health," "Homelessness," "Minority Health," and so on, including course syllabi, announcements of conferences, publications, and organizations.

APPENDIX B

SOME THOUGHTS

ON TEACHING

At least twice a year since 1989 I have cotaught two graduate seminars, one on poverty and health in the United States, the other on health in the developing world. I have had several partners in this project, most notably anthropologists Dan Perlman and Kira Foster. In my opinion, both Dan and Kira are gifted teachers, and much of what follows represents their thinking. We teach both at the University of California's health science campus in San Francisco (UCSF), and at the School of Public Health at the University of California Berkeley.

The format and content of the seminars was greatly influenced by what led up to them. For the preceding five years, I had held a teaching grant from the University of California Institute on Global Conflict and Cooperation. With this grant, several medical colleagues and I were teaching a course in the medical school called "The Health Professional and Nuclear War." I was growing less and less satisfied with this course. For one thing, the threat of nuclear war began to seem less urgent after the signing of the INF Treaty in 1987 and the fall of the Berlin Wall in 1989. For another thing, it was becoming steadily clearer to me each year that the threat of war in general was really a symptom of a growing social disease—the disease of rampant human inequality and injustice.

However, I had never made this problem a focus of my academic career, and did not know where to begin to address it in my teaching. It was a stroke of good luck that in 1988 I met Dan Perlman, who was then a graduate student in medical anthropology at UCSF. Perlman had already spent about seven years studying problems of social inequality and access to health care, and knew a great deal about it. He and I also shared an ethical and methodological point of view about teaching: that it must be value-based, and that the pedagogic methods must reinforce by demonstration the values we sought to convey.

Together, Perlman and I planned the pair of companion seminars. Our basic assumption was that health inequality can and should be greatly reduced by (1) distributing health and medical knowledge as widely as possible, thereby making it possible for underserved people to help themselves more effectively; (2) simultaneously empowering the underserved to address the economic and social inequalities that contribute to ill health—inequalities both between and within social classes. If communities can work together, we believe, people can make inroads against malnutrition, unsafe work, inadequate education, environmental hazards, and bad housing.

Given our assumptions about values and methods, the logical teaching method was to encourage the students' awareness of their own experiences of inequality, and empower them to take more control over their education. This should be done, moreover, within an atmosphere of shared responsibility and equal participation. Of course there is nothing revolutionary about this. We were—or I should say Dan was—already well aware of the methods of Paolo Freire, Miles Horton, and David Werner, whose works are cited elsewhere in this book. Our task was to adapt these methods to the specifics of our classes—the students' knowledge and experience base, the academic scheduling and logistic constraints, and the contents of our teaching.

Class Format

From the beginning, our classes have been very popular. I believe this was due at first to the novelty of what we were doing, and the enthusiasm that novelty inspired in both faculty and students. As the years have passed, the enterprise has become less novel for the teachers, and we have worked to keep the excitement alive in other ways. We have experimented carefully with format and content, and actively encouraged student feedback. We collect systematic class evaluations at the end of each term. The evaluations always contain a large majority of excellent ratings, which in itself only tells us that the sense of discovery and camaraderie in the classes remains high. We have not been able to stay in touch with most of our graduates, but those that we have followed seem to retain their commitment to community service, and to be able to put many of the ideas they learned into practice.

However, what follows here is not proposed as a formula for teaching this or any other topic. Rather, it is put forward as an example of an approach that seems to work pretty well. For one thing, other teachers will be working within other constraints of scheduling, class size, and student preparation.

Schedule and Student Characteristics

Our classes meet once a week, for two hours each meeting. At the medical school, the format is ten weeks. At the school of public health, it is fifteen weeks. The size of the class varies widely, but it seems to work best with around fifteen to twenty students. At the medical school, most of the participants are master's or doctoral students in nursing, preparing for careers as nurse practitioners, midwives, nursing administrators, or professors of nursing. There are often a few medical students and graduate social science students in these courses as well. In the school of public health, the participants range from undergraduates in a variety of majors, to preclinical medical students, to advanced graduates and even postdoctoral students in public health, including some experienced MDs. On the whole, we find the most experienced students tend to pull the skill level of the less experienced upward, rather than the other way around.

The classes always include a range of ethnicities. Students are U.S. born and foreign born of African, European, Middle Eastern, East and Southeast Asian, Pacific Island, and Latin American origin. We consider this diversity a great advantage of the classes, and encourage people to talk about their cultural experiences and points of view. Often the foreign-born students are among the most vocal and interesting in the class. There are of course cultural differences in communicative style, with foreign-born Africans and Asians tending to be less outspoken than the others. The use of student coleaders and journals, discussed below, are ways of maximizing participation of the less vocal students.

Since our seminars are elective rather than required, most of the students are drawn to the courses by a combination of interest in the topic and the reputation of the courses. I am aware that this makes our task much easier than that of teaching a required course. It not only puts a floor under the students' interest level, it also makes it possible for us to tell them not to take the course unless they really intend to participate fully and do their best.

Instructors

The course is always led by at least two instructors, with occasional support from expert visitors. Having a pair of teachers who work well as a team greatly improves the quality of the seminar. Each of us is able to notice nuances in both the content and the tone of the class discussion that the other has missed, and that need to be addressed. Also, good teaching requires a clear mind and a high energy level. Occasionally one of us is distracted or fatigued by other life events, and the other can usually help compensate for this.

We have experimented with various types and levels of instructor background. In addition to regular faculty and advanced graduate students, we have tried using community activists with little formal schooling. We sought out what I thought of as *living textbooks*—people whose personalities seemed to promise an active and challenging role in the class, and whose experience would lend a refreshingly personal and down-to-earth view of the problems we were discussing. These coteachers have included a South African nurse (Thandi Omobode), a former Mexican farmer turned health activist (Martin Bustos), an African American woman organizing her fellow welfare mothers for political advocacy (René Pecot), and two formerly homeless African American outreach workers from a local health access project (Lucille Anderson and Carla Roberts).

I still think the approach of including living textbooks is a promising one. They occasionally do jar the students out of their intellectual ruts by offering very distinct views of things, and they are often excellent resources when it comes to checking on the accuracy of generalizations and practicality of suggestions about the lives and health of the poor. There are difficulties, however, that have caused us to discontinue the experiment for now. The main problem is that the mutual lack of familiarity with one another's language and way of thinking simply makes it hard for graduate students and lay activists to join in an intellectual discussion, regardless of how much knowledge either one has of the topic. Participants on both sides of the academic divide must be able to follow the conversation fairly closely, join at the right moment, and craft their comments so that their counterparts can understand them.

So far, we have not been able to accomplish this well enough to continue with the lay instructors. It might be accomplished if one group or the other (students or lay instructors) could be trained in their counterparts' communicative style, but this would take more time and resources than we have. (At one point, we tried to get a grant to do just this, but were unsuccessful.) Other problems include the obstacles nonaffluent people often face when it comes to keeping appointments, and a certain diffidence that can overcome any of us when we find ourselves in very unfamiliar territory, such as a welfare mom on a university campus.

Our most effective instructors have had in common, then, (a) at least a university undergraduate level of academic training; (b) fairly good knowledge of sociology or cultural anthropology; and (c) a long-standing and strong dedication to human rights issues, including experience working with some low-income group somewhere. Experience in classroom teaching, while less necessary, also helps. Within this frame, we have found that students or professionals in nursing, medicine, anthropology, agricultural economics, psychology, or sociology can make excellent teachers using these methods. We also have students do some of the teaching—a point I will take up under "Participation," below.

Readings

Classroom discussion is supported by fifty to one hundred pages of assigned reading per meeting. This is absolutely essential. We organize the class into one-week "problem area" topics. At the first class meeting, we go over this reading list in detail, explaining the logic behind the choice and sequence of themes, and briefly characterizing the viewpoints, strengths, and weaknesses of the authors. We also emphasize the importance of doing the reading, and invite the students to critique the choice of topics and authors.

The most demanding aspect of the entire course for the instructor is to assemble readings that have the following characteristics:

- focus directly on at least some of the key issues under discussion,
- use language and concepts that are clear to students with varied interests and experience, and a broad range of disciplines,
- represent a wide range of opinion on the subject,
- represent a range of methods and purposes—for example, surveys, policy documents, news articles, ethnographies, and journalistic pieces.
- are not too long or too numerous.

For millennia (see *Ecclesiastes* 12:12) reading has been branded the great burden of higher education. Although my co-instructors and I are constantly trying to improve the reading list, we have found it impossible to assemble one that everybody likes, and have learned to settle for one that most students can stomach, and that provokes good discussion. I have also learned to take certain student prejudices with a grain of salt—especially the common misconception that any reading belongs in a history course if it is over five years old. Some of our best readings are over thirty years old. It helps of course to be able to locate, for the students, the author's place in the evolution of ideas on the topic.

Outside the Classroom: Meetings, E-mail, Journals

Three main methods are used to enrich and extend the classroom process: meetings, e-mail, and written journals. Students are encouraged to schedule meetings individually with faculty to talk about anything having to do with the class—further exploration of a question, help with an assignment, a problem with the format or content of the course, the relevance of the class to other work. This can be very helpful for instructors, as it gives a chance to explore each student's unique background and way of thinking. When I was commuting to the Berkeley campus from San Francisco, I had little opportunity to see the Berkeley students outside of class, and I scheduled half-hour coffee times with all of them to make up for this.

E-mail has proven to be a boon to teacher-student communication. Students can easily contact me with questions or suggestions. I can easily pass on information to the whole class, not only about assignments and logistics, but about ideas as well. Often, after having thought about a class discussion, it will occur to me that a crucial point was neglected, or that the class's reaction to an issue was not properly addressed. I can raise these issues in a collective e-mail before the discussion has gotten cold, and without taking up class time at the next meeting.

One year we had a particularly large class of about forty students. It was not one of the better classes, because there was not enough time for everyone to participate as much as they would have liked, but it led to an innovation that turned out to be very useful for classes of all sizes. We decided to have the students write down informally their thoughts about both the readings and the class discussions in a journal, which would be periodically handed in for our review and comment. Weekly journal entries of two or three pages were made mandatory, but we did not grade students on the contents. At first we wrote comments on the journals and handed them back two or three times per term. After several students remarked on how useful the comments were, we changed to handing back detailed comments on every weekly journal entry the following week.

The method taught us several new things. Some students who were very quiet in class had excellent ideas—ideas so good that we felt the need to incorporate them in the lessons. Some students wrote about powerful feelings aroused by the readings and discussions—feelings of sadness, anger, anxiety, helplessness. Clearly the class process had to be more sensitive to this dimension as well. Some students were struggling to understand the material. It represented a point of view so alien to their top-down, technocratic education that they did not know what to make of it. We had to think of intellectual bridges to get these students involved.

We have used these communication channels almost as much as the classroom itself, both as a teaching and as a learning tool. The classroom process that I will now describe is in part a product of this learning.

Process: Empowerment as Form and Content

If the methods I am proposing appear to be unusually demanding of time and energy, that is probably because I have spent years arranging things so that my coteachers and I are able to put a high priority on these classes compared with our other work. I don't know of any effective way of teaching these kinds of things that does not take strenuous commitment. The discussion of class process that follows makes this point still clearer, I think.

I have mentioned that from the beginning, we wanted the class format as well as the content to reflect the principle of empowerment as a way of mobilizing energy to improve health care. Chapters 7 and 8 of this book explain what I mean by empowerment, and why I think it is a useful way of looking at health care, especially as a way of opening access for those with limited power and resources.

Trust

Empowerment requires that all participants in the change process move toward active participation. This in turn requires that people set aside long-established doubts about their own effectiveness—something that can only happen in settings where they trust each other. At the beginning of the term, then, we are careful to establish an atmosphere of trust and openness in the classroom:

> (a) We have the students introduce themselves with a few words about their background and why they are taking the

class. This gives the instructors a chance to role model listening respectfully and showing interest in each person's presentation. It also demonstrates the principle that students' personal backgrounds and thoughts are important components of the class.

(b) We discuss the rules of interaction in the class, drawing attention to the need for mutual respect and sensitivity to feelings, and within this frame, for voicing opinions openly.

(c) Instructors regularly support students' comments by drawing attention to their interesting points. When a viewpoint is challenged either by the instructors or by a student, instructors are careful to give respect and support to those who have shown affinity for the challenged view. Occasionally heated discussions develop, in which the instructors become referees. As long as the atmosphere of trust holds up, these are among the most stimulating and instructive moments in the class.

(d) In class, instructors often reveal their own personal feelings and intellectual self-doubts, and admit their mistakes, setting a tone of openness and demonstrating that it is safe.

RESPONSIBILITY

Also at the beginning of the term, we tell the students that this is not a lecture class, but a participatory one. We are called instructors, but are actually facilitators of our own and others' learning, and the students are expected to take major responsibility for the direction and level of the discussion. We point out that this involves reading the discussion material thoroughly and critically, and coming to class with ideas about it.

To emphasize this point about shared responsibility, we let them know that the contents and format of the class are open, and they are free to change it any way they want, as long as there is a reasonable consensus for the change. In planning the schedule, we deliberately leave one to three meetings during the latter half of the semester open, without prescheduled topics. We tell the students to think about topics they would like to develop for these open meetings. Around the middle of the semester, the class chooses topics for the open meetings, and students volunteer to work with the instructors in finding readings, guest coleaders, and exercises for these topics. I will say more about this in the next section.

Critical feedback about the class is encouraged in various ways. In an empowerment framework, most students grow more confident about their opinions, and feel increasingly safe criticizing what they dislike. At any point during the term, if for any reason an instructor feels uncertain about the appropriateness of an assignment or a direction, the question is brought up with the students, either directly in class, or through the e-mail network.

RECOGNITION AND SUPPORT

I doubt that I have to say much about the need to recognize and support the individuality of each participant in the class. Commitment to a group process naturally flows from the feeling that one's unique personhood is recognized and accepted, and one's contributions valued. We learn and use everyone's name as early and as often as possible (even though I find this is a painfully difficult job). We take opportunities to refer in a friendly way to students' special traits (including mild and affectionate teasing where appropriate).

We try to demonstrate this respect for individuality in every interaction, not only in class, but out of it. Whenever possible, classroom seating is arranged around a large table or in a single large circle, with everyone (including the instructors) shoulder-to-shoulder rather than back-to-front. If space does not permit this, we approximate it as closely as possible, sometimes even sitting on the floor in preference to having tiers of participants. The worst possible classroom is one with files and rows of desks bolted to the floor.[1] People's non-intellectual needs, bodily and social, also deserve attention. When a student has a special problem, such as scheduling, we do our best to help them. In order to accommodate the calendars of busy nursing and medical students, we usually hold classes in the evening, when people tend to be a bit tired and hungry. Here, we have established a "potluck" tradition, where we, the instructors, supply soft drinks and juice, paper plates, napkins and glasses, and the students take turns bringing light snacks of crackers, raw vegetables and fruit, cookies or cake, or occasionally even a homemade casserole!

PARTICIPATION

Every single class has its stars and its wallflowers. We make a point of trying to broaden participation as much as possible, and have come up with several techniques. As I have already mentioned, e-mail and journals are among these, as is the subtle but steady effort to support self-esteem in the classroom. One method is to form breakout sessions where everyone has more freedom to be heard. Another method that the students especially like is to have class members take turns volunteering to colead sessions of the class. Still another is the open session, in which the students select an individual or committee who will completely plan a session.

Breakout sessions are by now a familiar method of increasing group participation. Often, a complex topic is broken down into components, and participants in the larger group elect which component they want to work on in a smaller group. Breakout sessions can be made of two or more people, up to about six or seven. Above that size, they tend to become too formal, and defeat their purpose, which is to give everyone ample time and self-confidence to talk. The concept is that in such a small group, people quickly get a feel for each other's personality and ideas. Leadership can be light and informal. The fact that each group is one of several gives it a sort of momentary identity, increasing members' motivation to contribute something unique to the larger class or conference. Breakout sessions usually have a record keeper, who reports back to the plenary group the results of their discussion. If the record keeper is skillful, he or she will make sure that the contributions of the quietest members are duly reported.

Student coleading is quite simple. At the beginning of the term, students are told that at the third meeting (by which time students have begun to feel more confident about their role in the class) a list of class sessions will be circulated, and that each of them is to sign up to colead at least one session. We explain the process: At the end of each class session, the student or students who have signed up to colead the next session, plus at least one instructor, will meet briefly to pick a time before the next class when they can all meet to form an agenda for that class. The volunteers are to do the reading and formulate discussion topics before this meeting, which usually takes place about an hour before the class itself. Depending on the size of the class and the enthusiasm of the students, each session might be led by as few as one, or as many as four students.

At the meeting, students offer their ideas about points of discussion for the class. Together with the instructor, they come up with an *A* list and a *B* list of discussion questions—the latter to be held in reserve in case their is extra time (which there virtually never is). The process often generates questions that the instructors would not have thought of. However, the experience and intuition of the instructors is crucial in helping decide which questions will fly. The group also roughs out a schedule of activities: what the sequence of issues will be, who will introduce each topic, how much time will be spent on it, and what format the discussion of each issue will take—plenary or breakout sessions, team debates, role plays, and so on.

When the class convenes, the instructors introduce the session leaders, who are by now known by the rest of the class, and pass the mantle of leadership to them. The dynamics of the classes are such that the students generally warm quickly to the discussion questions, and the time passes all too quickly. Each discussion has a dynamic of its own, and it is not unusual for this dynamic to lead the content far afield from the original agenda. The student coleaders and instructors have the option of letting it go or trying to bring it back, and here of course no firm rules can be written. It pays to be flexible up to a point, but identifying the point of intervention is, in our practice, pure art. I will return to this when I discuss the chemistry of classes.

The open session method is similar to the student coleader method, but gives students more responsibility, and can be encouraging to students who have expertise in a topic that does not appear on the original syllabus. As I mentioned earlier, we usually leave one or more of the later sessions of the syllabus blank for this purpose. We ask at the beginning of the class that students think about what topics they would like to cover in the blank sessions, and about three weeks beforehand, we devote about a half hour of class time to discussion of this question. Usually there are more good suggestions than open sessions, and the students have to vote on their favorites. Once a topic is selected, volunteers are recruited to work on it, and together they form a committee that works outside class hours to round up the readings, audiovisuals, or speakers, plan the agenda, and conduct the class. Instructors usually meet with the committee at least once before the event, so as to at least assuage our anxiety about what will happen. Some of the student-planned sessions have been among the all-time best.

PROCESS PROBLEMS

Thanks to the self-selected nature of the classes, and the emphasis on their social process, we have had amazingly few problems making them work smoothly. I will mention four recurrent ones: class size, class composition, the problem student, and runaway emotions.

Since the classes are electives in a large university, and since there are no prerequisites for them, it is difficult to predict how many students will want to take them. We have had classes with as many as thirty students and as few as ten that turned out quite well, but usually the limits of a good class seem to be between twelve and twenty-five, with an ideal of around fifteen to twenty. Thirty-five or forty does not work well, nor does less than ten. There needs to be enough energy and diversity on any given day to generate a lively discussion, and enough intimacy for people to develop a sense of trust and belonging. Occasionally we have been able by recruiting to build up an initial class of seven or eight to ten or more. When the initial class size is too big, we try to encourage the less enthusiastic members to switch to other classes, but not knowing a fair principle for excluding aspirants, and lacking the resources to run more than one section in a given term, we have never fully solved the problem of the occasional oversized class.

Class composition is rarely a problem, but twice we have encountered small classes in which virtually no one had the background needed to produce dynamic discussions. Our natural impulse in these situations is to spend a lot more time explaining the material to the students in class. This of course further dampens the empowerment dynamic, and is not a good solution. If it happens again, I believe the best approach will be to give the students more structured discussion assignments at first: encourage each one of them to develop a mini-expertise on that small facet of the day's topic that they find most interesting, so that the classroom energy continues to come from the students themselves.

It is a common experience in teaching student-centered seminars that one or more of the participants may be chronically disruptive of the process. By this I do not mean that their opinions are odd or unpopular, or that they stir up controversy, or that the instructor or some other students dislike them—such students can be the very fuel that drives a class to think. Rather, I mean those who show insensitivity to the needs of the class. They talk too much, or they often break the rules of respect, or they chronically ignore the direction of the discussion to pursue some private hobby horse, or they habitually introduce disruptive emotions like boredom or disgust that sap the flow of interaction. Sometimes the disruption results simply from a forceful personality, an arsenal of strong opinions, or a lack of insight about one's effect on the class. If so, a tactful one-on-one talk with the student outside of class is in order. We have been able to turn such problem students into allies by helping them to understand what kind of process we are trying to achieve in the class: one where controversy is welcome, as long as everyone has an equal chance to be heard, and no one feels threatened or disrespected by anyone else. In one case (and I would not prescribe this for everyone), we got a problem student to tape record the classes and then listen to her own performance with a critical ear. It worked, and I think it helped her career considerably in the long run.

Occasionally, though, the problem student is driven less by lack of social skill than by hostility. This will of course become clear when reasonable approaches to solve the problem fail. Such a situation can be absolutely deadly for this type of course, and has to be dealt with. I personally have great difficulty relating to hostile people, and my preference is to request help from a neutral third party if I cannot tolerate a student's behavior in class. Most universities have an officer—perhaps the dean of students—whose job description includes this kind of work. Admittedly, one occasionally meets students whose hostile agenda is so intractable that anything you do will be held against you, but there I can only say, don't give up without a damn good fight.

The best thing about our classes is that people become emotionally involved in both the issues and the learning process itself. Several students have written to tell us that a class changed their lives. This, of course, can also be a difficulty. Allowing themselves to open up emotionally leaves students highly vulnerable to disturbing feelings as well—guilt, shame, anxiety, even love. We rarely have tears in class, but it can happen (and has happened to me). The supportive atmosphere of the class usually helps people work through these feelings, and I have already mentioned the use of contact outside of class (meetings, e-mail, journals) to further deal with them. The instructor who uses this process, though, must be careful to warn students about negative feelings, and to give them a chance to express these. To my knowledge we have never had an emotional "casualty," in the sense that anyone had major or long-lasting upset as a result of it.

And I have to say something about flirting. In an atmosphere of emotional openness, erotic feelings can come to the fore also. Sometimes they can be pretty powerful. In my view, what students do about this among themselves is strictly their own business (as long as they don't do it in class!). They will make it their business in any case. It goes without saying that instructors must never become sexually involved with students, no matter whose idea it is.[2] Nevertheless, at the very least some passionate glances are going to sneak their way in and around the classroom, and a well-prepared instructor has thought about how to be ethical and considerate should he or she become involved as glancee, glancer, or both. Craft your own protocol. Self-awareness, a sense of pathos, and the background of a stable and satisfying love life can all be invaluable.

Measuring Success: The Chemistry of Classes

A highly successful student-centered class is easy to distinguish from a less successful one. In the better classes a rapport develops among all the participants, so that they clearly enjoy being together for the purpose at hand. Virtually all the students read thoroughly, think clearly, and show high energy in the classroom. Whether the mood is somber or hilarious, it is usually intense, and seems to bring people closer together. Many of the students want to do more than the assignments. Some of them want to continue studying the issues, or continue meeting one another, after the class is finished. People change noticibly in the course of a semester. They become more self-confident and more self-critical. Their speaking and listening skills improve. It is an intoxicating experience for the teacher.

Unfortunately, not all classes are like this. The least successful ones are just . . . classes. Students usually do the assignments, and learning does take place. Many of the participants enjoy the nurturant teaching style and rate the class highly. But the discussions have a mechanical quality, as though this were a gym class going through mental calisthenics. A bright insight may flare up, only to be allowed to fade away. The energy level is fairly low. At the end, the students politely thank us for our efforts and go about their lives, probably relatively unchanged. Some classes are only moderately successful. They have peaks and troughs of energy, they produce a few high-fliers who leave the others behind.

Truly sharing power with a new group of students every few months is a risky business, one that offers a teacher long periods of frustration as well as triumph. No matter how well prepared one is, one cannot really predict or control the overall mood. Rather, each singular group of students seems fairly quickly to develop its own distinct and durable chemistry, pace, energy level, even shared self-image, that is difficult to influence. I do not know what the ingredients of this chemistry are. Some classes have a full complement of bright, well-trained participants, but never seem to take off. Others start with less but pull themselves up by their bootstraps and achieve a high level of energy and productivity. Some successful classes are culturally and experientially diverse, others not. If I had to identify the key ingredient of success I would say it is rapport—an easy mutual respect and feeling of kinship that both motivates students to contribute and frees them from their inhibitions and self-doubts. This chapter sets forth what we have learned in our efforts to nurture this rapport. But we have not yet learned how to conjure it in groups where it is not ready to emerge.

Content

It is not my aim to argue for or against any subject matter the reader might want to include in a student-centered seminar like ours. I believe the method lends itself well to any subject that touches on social justice and social change—a wide range indeed. In selecting content for a graduate course in the health sciences at least (the only arena where I can speak from much experience), I think there are four useful principles: knowledge of subject, knowledge of students, clarity of goals (that is, knowledge of self), and flexibility.

These four principles form a mutually supporting grid, as none is sound without the other. The more I know about poverty and the health of the poor, the clearer I can formulate what my students need to know about it, and set firm goals for a course. I must know what sorts of ideas and knowledge my students have in order to shape material so that their abilities and my goals will come together. I must also know what their work is like in order to formulate goals that address their needs. And since I cannot possibly teach everything of importance about the subject, I must decide what is most important, and build the content around that.

Flexibility enters at every point. As the teaching process unfolds, I learn about the students around me, and about students in general. My beliefs and values are often challenged in class, and I must rethink them. As knowledge of the subject deepens, new relevancies are revealed. Teaching is a bit like politics, it involves a set of goals and principles, a matrix of historical realities, and an ability to bring these together to effect change, by sensing the unfolding needs and moods of the participants. If a bit of content clearly misses the mark set by overall goals, change it there and then. If a student comes up with a strong suggestion, adopt it at once. If an insight reveals that your priorities were mistaken, rethink them the same day.

Summary

This brief word on student-centered learning doesn't convey the essence of it when it works, which is a feeling that one is changed by taking part. Neither do I expect that this description is enough of a guide to produce a good class. Perhaps readers who already have personal experience of what I am writing about can use this to verify and sharpen their ideas. Perhaps those who want such an experience will be encouraged to begin the long process of trial and error that brought my coteachers and me to where we are.

NOTES

CHAPTER 1 *Through the Telescope: Encountering Poverty*

1. In one particularly ironic case, the City of New York, whose public schools rank among the worst in the nation, spent $150 million to build a posh magnet high school for its smartest kids. The *Times* described the students as a "brainy bunch" that "*deserves* every bit of indulgence a cash-strapped city can muster" (Kozol 1996,153; emphasis mine). Academic talent now separates the deserving from the undeserving poor as well.

2 In the United States, normal cultural inconsistency is complicated to some extent by the diverse origins and ways of life of our people. Some anthropologists would say that I am stretching the concept of culture even to talk about American *norms*—that there is no typical American, and therefore no true American culture. I answer this with two observations. First, there is no *culture* of any kind, anywhere. Culture is an abstraction. It is simply a mental tool that allows us to think more systematically about the differences between social groups. To say that "Americans value individual autonomy," is just to make a generalization based on looking at the way Americans tend to behave, in comparison with Japanese and Zulus and Italians.

Second, such abstractions are not as tenuous as some might think. Given the size and heterogeneity of our country, it is surprising how similar and consistent are the lessons we all learn in school, and the messages we all get from TV, newspapers, advertising, films, and books. As one who has lived and traveled a good deal in Japan, Central America, and Europe, I am sometimes struck by the fear of controversy one finds in American public discourse, as compared with that of other countries. It is as if the very heterogeneity of our people makes our leaders want to seem as mainstream and as average as possible. In American politics, if you want to get really vicious about an opponent, you say she is "out of touch with the people," which is another way of saying her ideas are controversial. I will come back to this point when I discuss the treatment of poverty in the media.

3. *Time Magazine*, in a moment of self-consciousness, announced on September 1, 1997 (p. 25), that while the proportion of African Americans among the poor runs at 29 percent, the number of stories about poverty illustrated with pictures of African Americans in the leading newsweeklies runs at 62 percent.
4. Cost shifting is the practice of overcharging those who are insured or can pay for services, and applying the excess funds to the care of those who can pay less.

CHAPTER 5   *The Poor on the Picture Tube: The "Debates" on Welfare and Health Care Reform*

1. For a more thorough discussion of the role of symbolism in American politics, see George Lakoff's *Moral Politics* (1966). Lakoff argues that the political Left has failed to understand the symbolic structure of political beliefs, thereby conceding the power of unconscious manipulation to the Right. The Right alone, says Lakoff, understands that politics "is about the family."
2. The reader is referred to the rich literature on the concept, beginning with Machiavelli, and extending through Rousseau and Marx to Foucault and Bourdieu.

CHAPTER 7   *The Evolution and Role of Community Health Centers*

1. Like most jargon in health politics, the word is deliberately misleading. Ultimately, it is the consumers and the taxpayers who pay for health services *and* the enormous administrative costs and profits that go with them. The word *middlemen* would be accurate.
2. Another misnomer. What capitated payment systems do, and what they are meant to do, is manage money. Those who are required to make care decisions are simply told to do so within a given budget. This is not management.

CHAPTER 8   *Facilitating Community Involvement*

1. The work of German sociologist Georg Simmel on this problem is classic. Simmel notes that only in an intimate dyad can the individual be simultaneously "for himself" and "for the group." (Simmel 1950,137–138)

APPENDIX B   *Some Thoughts on Teaching*

1. One of our best classes at Berkeley fled such a room and became semi-nomadic, meeting in whatever vacant space they could commandeer for the day. We met in elegant boardrooms, musty basement laboratories, students' houses, and on campus lawns. The shared hardship actually seemed to strengthen the students' dedication to the class,

and when it was over, they continued to meet from time to time just for the fun of it.

2. I would prefer it if teachers made a general rule not to succumb to Cupid once the mentor relationship had ended, either. Otherwise, one can be tempted to begin counting the days until the formal relationship with a particular student ends, thereby pretty much defeating the purpose of the professional taboo. But I realize I would be condemning about half my colleagues with such a rule.

BIBLIOGRAPHY

Adams, F. 1975. *Unearthing Seeds of Fire: The Idea of Highlander*. Winston-Salem, N.C.: J. F. Blair.

Aday, L. A. 1993. *At Risk in America: The Health and Health Care Needs of Vulnerable Populations in the United States*. San Francisco: Jossey-Bass.

Adler, N., W. T. Boyce, M. A. Chesney, S. Folkman, and L. Syme. 1993. "Socioeconomic Inequalities in Health: No Easy Solution." *Journal of the American Medical Association* 269, no. 24:3140–3145.

Bagdikian, B. 1992. *The Media Monopoly*. 4th ed. Boston: Beacon Press.

Barlett, D. L., and J. B. Steele. 1992. *America: What Went Wrong?* Kansas City: Andrews and McMeel.

Bernstein, B. 1969. "Welfare in New York City." *City Almanac* (February): 120.

Bodenheimer, T., and K. Grumbach. 1995. *Understanding Health Policy: A Clinical Approach*. Stamford, Conn: Appleton and Lange.

Bourgois, Philippe. 1995. *In Search of Respect: Selling Crack in El Barrio*. Cambridge: Cambridge University Press.

Brown, L. 1997. "Ten Commandments of Community-based Research." In *Community Organizing and Community Building for Health*, edited by M. Minkler. New Brunswick, N.J.: Rutgers University Press.

Brown, S., and L. Eisenberg, eds. 1995. *The Best Intentions: Unintended Pregnancy and the Well-being of Children and Families*. Washington, D.C.: National Academy Press.

Census Bureau. 1998. *Poverty: 1997 Highlights*. Washington, D.C.: U.S. Census Bureau.

Cooper, M. 1997. "When Push Comes to Shove: Who Is Welfare Reform Really Helping?" *Nation*, 2 June, 11–15.

Couto, R. A. 1982. *Streams of Idealism and Health Care Innovation*. New York: Columbia University Press.

———. 1991. *Ain't Gonna Let Nobody Turn Me Round*. Philadelphia: Temple University Press.

Daniel, M. 1999. "Health Center's Bankruptcy Puts Neighborhood Care at Risk." *Boston Globe*. Internet ed., 31 January.

DeParle, J. 1994. "Better Work than Welfare, But What If There's Neither?" *New York Times Magazine*, 18 December, 44ff.

Doyal, L. 1979. *The Political Economy of Health*. London: Pluto Press.

Duff, R. S., and A. B. Hollingshead. 1968. *Sickness and Society*. New York: Harper and Row.

Duggar, B., B. Balicki, and A. Zuvekas. 1981. *Costs and Utilization Patterns for Comprehensive Health Center Users*. Washington, D.C.: Bureau of Primary Health Care, U.S. Department of Health and Human Services.

Dunn, K. 1994. "The Politics of Fear: The Recent Hysteria over Violent Crime Is Based More on Myth than Genuine Danger." *San Francisco Chronicle*. This World Section, 12 June, 7–12.

Dutton, D. B. 1986. "Social Class, Health, and Illness." In *Applications of Social Science to Clinical Medicine and Health Policy* edited by L. Aiken and D. Mechanic. New Brunswick, N.J.: Rutgers University Press.

Fitchen, J. M. 1981. *Poverty in Rural America: A Case Study*. Boulder, Colo.: Westview Press.

Frankl, V. 1959. *Man's Search for Meaning*. New York: Touchstone.

Freeman, H. K., J. Kiecolt, and H. M. Allen. 1982. *Community Health Centers: An Initiative of Enduring Utility*. Washington, D.C.: Bureau of Primary Health Care, U.S. Department of Health and Human Services.

Freeman, W. 1987. "Responsibility in COPC: An Analysis in Medical Ethics." In *Community Oriented Primary Care*, edited by Paul Nutting. Albuquerque: University of New Mexico.

Freire, P. 1970. *Cultural Action for Freedom*. Cambridge, Mass.: Harvard Educational Review.

Frobel, F., J. Heinrichs, and O. Kreye. 1977. "The Tendency Towards a New International Division of Labor." *Review* 1 no. 1:73–88.

Gans, H. 1963. *The Urban Villagers*. New York: Basic Books.

Gautam, K., B. Arrington, and C. Campbell. 1995. "Inner City Hospitals: A Call for Research." *Journal of Health Care for the Poor and Underserved* 6 no. 4:387–402.

Gingrich, N. 1994. *The Contract with America*. New York: Times Books.

Ginsberg, N. 1993. "Sweden: The Social-Democratic Case." In *Comparing Welfare States: Britain in International Context*, edited by A. Cochrane and J. Clarke. London: Sage.

Grossman, M., and D. Goldman. 1982. *An Economic Analysis of Community Health Centers*. Washington, D.C.: Bureau of Primary Health Care, U.S. Department of Health and Human Services.

Hawkins, D. 1993. "Inequality, Culture, and Interpersonal Violence." *Health Affairs* (winter): 80–95.

HCFA (Health Care Financing Administration). 1998. "Managed Care in Medicare and Medicaid," *HCFA Fact Sheet*, 20 February.

Hess, B. 1991. "Growing Old in America in the 1990s." In *Growing Old in America*, edited by B. Hess and E. W. Markson. 4th ed. New Brunswick, N.J.: Transaction Books.

Howell, J. T. 1973. *Hard Living on Clay Street: Portraits of Blue Collar Families*. Garden City, New York: Anchor Books.

Kappeler, V., M. Blumer, and G. Potter. 1996. *The Mythology of Crime and Criminal Justice*. Prospect Heights, Ill.: Waveland Press.

Katz, M. 1989. *The Undeserving Poor*. New York: Pantheon.

———. 1995. *Improving Poor People*. Princeton: Princeton University Press.

Kiefer, C. 1974. *Changing Cultures, Changing Lives*. San Francisco: Jossey Bass.

Kilborn, P. 1998. "Cutting the Poor and the Elderly: A Managed-Care Retreat." *New York Times*, 6 July, A1.

Kotlowitz, A. 1991. *There Are No Children Here*. New York: Anchor Books.

Kozol, J. 1995. *Amazing Grace: The Lives of Children and the Conscience of a Nation*. New York: Crown Books.

Lakoff, G. 1996. *Moral Politics: What Conservatives Know That Liberals Don't*. Chicago: University of Chicago Press.

Lewis, O. 1959. *Five Families: Mexican Case Studies in the Culture of Poverty*. New York: Basic Books.

Liebmann, G. W. 1995. "Addressing Illegitimacy: The Root of Real Welfare Reform." *Heritage Foundation Backgrounder* 1032.

Luft, H. S. 1978. *Poverty and Health: Economic Causes and Consequences of Health Problems*. Cambridge, Mass.: Ballinger.

Mansbridge, J. 1973. "Time, Emotion and Inequality: Three Problems of Participatory Groups." *Journal of Applied Behavioral Science* 9 no. 2/3:351–368.

NACHC (National Association of Community Health Centers). 1996. *America's Health Centers: Quick Facts*. Washington, D.C.: NACHC.

Nakao, A. 1997. "Welfare Becomes Workfare, As Society Changes." *San Francisco Chronicle*, 2 February.

Nutting, P., ed. 1990. *Community-Oriented Primary Care*. Albuquerque: University of New Mexico Press.

Oster, S., E. Lake, and C. Oksman. 1979. *The Definition and Management of Poverty*. Vol. 1. Boulder, Colo.: Westview Press.

Perucci, C., E. Rapiti, D. Porta, F. Forastiere, and D. Fusco. 1999. "Socioeconomic Inequalities of Survival of People with AIDS before and after the Introduction of the Highly Effective Antiretroviral Therapy." Paper presented at the Ninth Annual Public Health Forum, London School of Hygiene and Tropical Medicine, London, April 20, 1999.

Piven, F., and R. Cloward. 1971. *Regulating the Poor*. New York: Random House.

Rector, R. 1995. "Why Congress Must Reform Welfare." *Heritage Foundation Backgrounder* 1063:1–12.

Relman, A. S. 1986. "The Physician's Role in Preventing Nuclear War." *New England Journal of Medicine* 315 no. 14:889–890.

Rosenberg, C. E. "Social Class and Medical Care in Nineteenth Century America: The Rise and Fall of the Dispensary." *Journal of the History of Medicine and Allied Sciences* 29:32–54.

Rosenthal, M. G. 1994. "Single Mothers in Sweden: Work and Welfare in the Welfare State." *Social Work* 39 no. 3:270–279.

Sanders, D., and R. Carver. 1985. *The Struggle for Health*. London: Macmillan.

Sardell, A. 1988. *The U.S. Experiment in Social Medicine: The Community Health Center Program, 1965–1986.* Pittsburgh: University of Pittsburgh Press.

Schiller, B. 1974. "Want Ads and Jobs for the Poor." *Manpower* (January).

———. 1984. *The Economics of Poverty and Discrimination.* Englewood Cliffs, N. J.: Prentice Hall.

Schubiner, H., R. Scott, and A. Tzelepis. 1993. "Exposure to Violence among Inner-city Youths." *Journal of Adolescent Health* 14:214–221.

Schwartz, J., and T. Volgy. 1993. "Above the Povery Line, But Poor." *Nation*, 3 February, 191–192.

Sigerist, H. 1929. "The Special Position of the Sick." In *Henry E. Sigerist on the Sociology of Medicine*, edited by M. I. Roemer. New York: MD Publications, 1960.

Simmel, G. 1909. "The Poor." In *Poverty: Power and Politics*, edited by C. Waxman. New York: Grosset and Dunlap.

———. 1950. *The Sociology of Georg Simmel.* Translated and edited by Kurt Wolff. New York: Free Press.

Smolensky, E., E. Evenhouse, and S. Reilly. 1995. *Welfare Reform in California.* Berkeley: Institute of Governmental Studies, University of California.

Stack, C. 1975. *All Our Kin.* New York: Harper and Row.

Starfield, B., N. R. Powe, J. R. Weiner, M. Stuart, D. Steinwachs, S. H. Schoole, and A. Gerstenberger. 1994. "Costs versus Quality in Different Types of Primary Health Care Settings." *Journal of the American Medical Association* 272 no. 24:1903–1908.

Starr, P. 1982. *The Social Transformation of American Medicine.* New York: Basic Books.

Stepick, A., and G. Grenier. 1993. "Cubans in Miami" In *In the Barrios: Latinos and the Underclass Debate*, edited by J. Moore and R. Pinderhughes. New York: Russell Sage.

Stevens, J. E. 1994. "Myths of Violence." *San Francisco Chronicle.* This World Section, 12 June , 10.

Stringer, Ernest. 1996. *Action Research: A Handbook for Practitioners.* Thousand Oaks, Calif.: Sage.

Syme, S. L., and L. F. Berkman. 1976. "Social Class, Susceptibility, and Sickness." *American Journal of Epidemiology* 104:1–8.

Turiel, J. 1995. "Interviews with Founders of the Over 60 Health Center." Unpublished manuscript by author. Berkeley, Calif.

Veatch, R. M. 1981. *A Theory of Medical Ethics.* New York: Basic Books.

Walter, C. 1997. "Community Building Practice: A Conceptual Framework." In *Community Organizing and Community Building for Health*, edited by M. Minkler. New Brunswick, N.J.: Rutgers University Press.

Ware, J. E., M. S. Bayliss, W. H. Rogers, M. Kosinski, and A. R. Tarlov. 1996. "Differences in Four-Year Outcomes for Elderly and Poor Chronically Ill Patients Treated in HMO and Fee-for-Service Systems." *Journal of the American Medical Association* 276 no. 13:1039–1047.

Weiner, J. M., and E. Engel. 1991. *Improving Access to Health Services for Children and Pregnant Women.* Washington, D.C.: Bureau of Primary Health Care, U.S. Department of Health and Human Services.

Weinreb, L. F., and E. L. Bassuk. 1990. "Health Care of Homeless Families: A Growing Challenge for Family Medicine." *Journal of Family Practice* 31 no. 1:74–80.

Wellstone, P. 1999. "America's Disappeared." *Nation*, 12 July, 5–6.

Wilson, M. 1993. "The German Welfare State: A Conservative Regime in Crisis." In *Comparing Welfare States: Britain in International Context*, edited by A. Cochrane and J. Clarke. London: Sage.

Yee, D. L., and J. A. Capitman. 1996. "Health Care, Access, Health Promotion, and Older Women of Color." *Journal of Health Care for the Poor and Underserved* 7 no. 3:252–272.

INDEX

ABOUT THE AUTHOR

Christie W. Kiefer is professor of anthropology in the department of anthropology, history, and social medicine, University of California School of Medicine, San Francisco, and a member of the board of directors of Lifelong Medical Care, a group of six community-owned clinics in Alameda County, California. Kiefer's other writings are on East Asian and Asian American cultures, aging, primary health care in developing countries, and violence and war.